The French Twist

Twelve Secrets of
Decadent Dining and
Natural Weight
Management

The French Twist

Carol Cottrill, CNC

NEW YORK

The French Twist

Published by:
Morgan James Publishing
The Entrepreneurial Publisher
5 Penn Plaza, 23rd Floor
New York City, New York 10001
(212) 655-5470 Office
(516) 908-4496 Fax
www.MorganJamesPublishing.com

Cover Design by:
Stacy Claywell
Claywell Design

Illustration by:
Jacqueline Bissett

ISBN 978-1-61448-166-9 Hard cover
ISBN 978-1-61448-162-1 Paperback
ISBN 978-1-61448-163-8 eBook

Library of Congress Control Number: 2011943481

The information contained in this book should not be a substitute for the advice of the reader's personal physician or other medical professional.

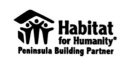

In an effort to support local communities, raise awareness and funds, Morgan James Publishing donates a percent of all book sales for the life of each book to Habitat for Humanity Peninsula and Greater Williamsburg.
Get involved today, visit www.HelpHabitatForHumanity.org

So often times it happens that we live
our lives in chains.
And we never even know we have the key.

—Eagles, "Already Gone"

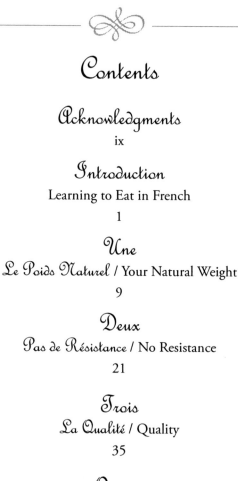

Contents

Acknowledgments

To begin, I'd like to acknowledge my clients, whose courage, determination, and trust make my work so meaningful for me. Everything I know, I have learned from you. To those whose experiences appear in this book under French aliases—I am so grateful. Your stories are a significant contribution.

To my Americans abroad, Carolyn Murphy, Susan Warsaw, and Amanda Sosa-Stone, whose personal experiences brighten these pages—*merci beaucoup!*

Josh Freidland, please accept my sincere appreciation for allowing me to share moments from your roundtable discussion with Pascale Weeks, Clotilde Dusoulier, Estelle Tracy, and Requia Badr. This book was enriched by their French twist.

To Marc David, Alton Brown, and Alan Cohen—you have helped me advance my knowledge in all things food and beyond. Thank you for your insight.

Allow me to recognize a wonderful literary agent—Kristina Holmes, who introduced me to David Hancock, founder of Morgan James Publishing. Kristina you are some matchmaker—it was love at first sight.

Which leads me to my admiration for David Hancock, who in our first meeting embraced this book's potential and the importance of its message. David, I am eternally grateful to you and everyone at Morgan James Publishing for making my dream come true.

For her prized creative direction I extend my gratitude to Stacy Claywell. Stacy, your flair for design and beauty coupled with gentle and reassuring oversight are an author's dream. *Je vous remercie de tout coeur.*

To Jacqueline Bissett—with the stroke of your brush *The French Twist* came to life. One of my wisest decisions was selecting you as my cover illustrator. Cheers!

To my PR professional extraordinaire, Cristina Calvet-Harrold—what a platform you have created, and what a friend you have become. Thank you from the bottom of my heart.

To my family and friends, who played an invaluable part in the outcome of this book—who read my work in the roughest form and offered me suggestions, reassurance, and support. I am most grateful.

A special thank-you to my cousin Trish Doyle, who took on the role of chief researcher without being asked, and my sister-in-law, Lynn Bowen, who blessed me with her unceasing love and encouragement. I appreciate you both so very much.

To my parents, who fed me lovingly, thank you for a balanced approach to eating and an incredible sweet tooth. To my son Richie Hayes, who dodged the sweet tooth, thanks for sharing my love of words and reading.

To my closest friend, Marisa Bryniarski, who has been a one-person cheering squad for me for more than thirty years. You never doubted my success for a moment. No one has ever had a better friend.

Finally, the most heartfelt affection and appreciation to the two people who have been by my side as this project evolved, providing unconditional encouragement and support. I could write an entire book describing their acts of love and commitment, but since at least one of them will have to edit this, I shall refrain.

Patricia Fogarty, my editor. We met as I stared down a rough outline of 10,000 words. You are an editor equipped with mind reading and coaching know-how galore. Your suggestions and edits resulted in exactly the book I wanted to write. You are so much more than my editor—you are my teacher, my shrink, and my dear, dear friend. There are no words adequate enough to thank you for being you.

John Cottrill, my husband. No one has ever cared for me in the way that you do. Not once during the writing of this manuscript did your belief and enthusiasm for the successful outcome of this book wane. Your guidance, love, and encouragement have enabled me to make a significant difference in my life as well as the lives of others. It is the greatest blessing of my life to have you as mine. ❧

Learning to Eat in French

I STUDIED THE FRENCH LANGUAGE with a tutor, repeated Rosetta Stone an embarrassing number of times, and endured private lessons and lots of homework from a Swiss teacher who swore her native tongue of Schweizerdeutsch would not affect the French pronunciation I struggled to master. I watched every French movie with English subtitles ever made and fell in love with actor Daniel Auteuil along the way, which proved to be the most enjoyable of the methods.

In the end, after hundreds of dollars and thousands of hours, here are the words that have become the core of my French vocabulary:

croissant

baguette

ménage à trois
(a threesome of desserts)

chocolat

macaron

boulangerie

bon appétit!

It turns out that language and customs take time to learn, but the discovery of a country's food is really the most efficient way to embrace a culture. And Americans are all about efficiency, so instead of speaking my way through France when I visited in 2007, I dined my way through.

My strategy on this trip to France—the first with *mon amour* John, my husband of one year—was to pursue a holy trinity of sorts, a feast we relished three times a day. No grazing or convenience foods on the run, no snacking, no metabolically ordained five mini-meals, no protein shakes, absolutely nothing that resembled my normal routine. You see, I am an American nutritionist—a control freak who knows everything about calories, carbohydrates, intake, output, and, so I thought, weight management.

The average weight of the adult Frenchwoman, who is just over
5 feet 3 inches tall, is 137.6 pounds,* while in the United States
the average weight for adult women is 164.7 pounds.*
Even adjusting for the slight difference in average height—
here we're just under 5 feet 4 inches—we're a heftier and
thus probably unhealthier bunch than our French counterparts.

This visit with John was not my first experience of France. That was in 1998, when a good friend and I took a side trip after completing a business assignment in Belgium. The diet du jour was low carb, and I was consuming lots of lean protein. Imagine what fun that was in the land of *haute cuisine!* I allowed myself one yeast-leavened, sweet Belgian waffle served up hot at the Brussels train station just before boarding the Eurostar for Paris. If I hadn't been on a speeding train that quickly reached 125 miles an hour, I would have jumped off for another of those tasty treats. My only faux pas on that trip to Europe was that one waffle. While in Paris, no delicate crêpe, no crusty baguette, not even a little muesli passed my lips. I remained a self-righteous, protein-eating example for the rest of the visit. "What's up with the skinny bread and butter eating French women?" I wondered.

---

* The Notes section at the end of the book contains citations of sources for material marked with an asterisk.

The next time I traveled to Paris was just a few months later; my trendy diet was now low-carb *and* dairy-free. I was just beginning my studies in nutrition, and all the talk about humans being the only mammals to drink the milk of another animal was getting to me. In case my language skills didn't suffice, I carried a little note written in French that explained my desire to avoid dairy products. I passed it to every waiter and continued to wonder why the French have a disparaging view of Americans. Anyway, I'm not sure what is worse, a lack of baguette or the absence of Brie, but my guess is that in France dismissing bread and avoiding cheese are considered equally stupid. Yet again, I took pride in and had a sense of superiority about my diet. "What's up with the happy, lactose-tolerant French women?" I wondered.

My third trip to France in 1999 was not the charm, although at the time I considered myself lucky to be in Nice for the Cannes Film Festival, where there were plenty of wonderful choices that fit into my eating plan. By this time I was deep into my nutritional studies. I enjoyed a day off when the film festival concluded and headed straight for the beach, toting my schoolbooks. I quickly spied a topless middle-aged woman. Her shoulders were thrown back so far that the blades nearly touched one another; her torso lunged forward, her breasts flopped to her waist like shrunken torpedoes, and her hands were placed solidly on her hips. In an effort to take in the maximum amount of sun, she rolled her head back and, with her eyes closed, relished the day. All over the beach, topless women of every age and shape were just as comfortable. "What's up with the unrestricted freedom of the French women?" I wondered.

THE REAL FRENCH PARADOX

The average life expectancy in France is 81. The average
life expectancy in the United States is 78.1 years of age.
Did someone say croissant?*

Love changes everything. The journey to Paris in 2007 with John was a continuation of the life we'd begun together, a union of love, contentment, and more happiness than I have ever known. The need to distract myself with a diet du jour or to control my food had vanished. In its absence I found equilibrium, peace, freedom, and satiety.

For the first time I was able to fully digest all that Paris had to offer, beginning with *le petit déjeuner*, then *le déjeuner*, then *le goûter*, and ultimately *le dîner*. Plus I no longer concerned myself with the inability to utter a word that any real French person would understand. Instead my motto became, "When in France if you can't speak it—eat it!"

It was at the airport, as we waited for our return flight, that I first noticed that my skinny Prada pants, generally reserved for the days following a week or two with the flu, were loose. Maybe they had stretched—that had to be it. There's no way I could have lost weight considering the decadence I had indulged in. *Au contraire*—I had lost weight, and so had John!

Within the pages of this book I will unravel the French Paradox, which of course is no paradox at all. It's a dilemma, yes, and French women heed the wisdom of twelve secrets that keep them enjoying food, life, family, and friends to the fullest. And while there are secrets, there is no magic, black or white, when it comes to weight management. Our bodies don't betray us—we betray our bodies, and the biggest betrayal begins with the latest fad diet.

The French know that, like history, mealtime repeats itself. In contrast, the American mania for dieting leaves us with a deep-seated fear that we're not getting enough food, and in response we overeat, devouring what we perceive to be our "last supper" over and over and over again.

So why not give your attitudes about food a French twist? In adopting *la manière française*, you may not learn to speak the language, but you will find and maintain your natural, healthy weight effortlessly. And you will rejoice in the mind and body that result when you feed them only healthy ideas and the highest-quality food.

WHO'S THE FATTEST OF THEM ALL?

The United States holds the number 1 position out of 30 countries. Americans enjoy the dubious distinction of having the highest obesity ranking in the world—34.3 percent of our population weighs in as obese. France lags behind, at 24th— only 10.5 percent of the French population is obese.*

Don't get me wrong—I love being an American. A peanut butter and banana sandwich is one of my favorite meals. I believe it should be mandatory to eat a hotdog at the ballpark, a chocolate chip cookie fresh from the oven, and lots of homemade apple pie. We Americans are more the informal *tu* than the formal *vous*, and I wouldn't want it any other way; my girlfriends spill their troubles at the drop of a hat—something a French girl would never do. Levis and Hanes suit me better than *haute couture*, although you'll never get between me and a Chanel handbag!

But . . . when it comes to dining and weight management, the French have it figured out. We Americans buy a heck of a lot of diet books and surround ourselves with even more potions and exercise paraphernalia, not to mention the hours of time we devote to the cause—yet all the while we and, most important, our children become more obese by the day.

Maybe the answer lies in simply noticing the differences and values of our two cultures and changing it up a bit. I fully intend to enjoy my peanut butter sandwich, and I may even do so while standing and watching *Dancing with the Stars*. But I'll also be sure to include the tried-and-true customs of the French in order to discover the perfect balance of eating French, American style.

Connecting the Dots

I've been told that in order to effectively write about a topic one first must gain perspective on the subject matter. I suppose that's why it has taken me so long to put this book together. Since I first had the impulse, I've accumulated years of personal experience and, through my work as a nutritionist, knowledge of the eating habits— and the related joys and miseries—of many other people. Good experiences, as well as some not so good ones, have been an essential part of my education and growth.

I could not have written this book ten years ago, although I dreamed of doing so. Still, all the while—sometimes in the back of my mind, other times at the front—I remained faithful in my quest to cut through the negative aspects of the dieting mentality for something better, something *natural*. I craved freedom, peace, balance, and nourishment, both physically and emotionally. I knew others did as well.

On my journey I have been greatly rewarded with glimpses of enlightenment that encouraged me to stay the course. As the latest and greatest diets came and went, magazine articles and books featuring diets of deprivation filled my trash bin. When I muted television spots featuring instant gratification and quick-fix promises, a growing luminosity allowed me to see the path that was opening before me. The brightness was finally radiant enough to bring me to this point in time.

WE ARE ALL THE SAME

It was during the late 1980s that I developed an attraction to and interest in other cultures while hosting foreign exchange students through the American Field Service. I count the time I spent with these young people as some of the most profound, life-altering, and insight-generating periods of my life. Daniela (Dani) from Germany, Tomoko from Japan, Bernhard (Bernie) from Austria, and Carl from France are responsible for the curiosity, love, and admiration I feel for the people and customs of other countries.

I remain grateful for this special gift—an up-close and personal perspective on other people and cultures—from my foreign exchange children. Their diverse lives and traditions forever opened my eyes and heart to cultures beyond my own. In embracing their lives and our differences, I learned about something more important—our similarities. It's fair to say that my appetite for all things French was cultivated while studying the behaviors and practices of my unguarded overseas students.

Bernie's favorite seat in our house in the suburbs of Chicago was at the kitchen counter. There we shared stories and secrets, like the time Bernie confessed that he exaggerated his accent because the American girls loved to hear him speak. Together we baked a cake, Bernie translating the directions on the box he had carried all the way from Austria, then reading the German aloud as I stirred the batter.

There's just something about a sixteen-year-old kid who's enjoying baking a cake with his host mom that warms my heart to this day. Simple moments like this reassure me that, no matter where we originate, in the end we are all the same. When we combine our mutual desires with our diverse traditions, we are able to whip up the perfect cake or the ideal soufflé—warm, fluffy, and delicious.

Mine is not a radical story; it's probably not very different from your own. The covert messages we all receive every day of our lives, starting when we first begin to observe our surroundings, are similar. For many people, including a disproportionate number of women, these external messages can become problematic. Often they lead us away from developing a true sense of self and toward a dependence on everything and everyone except our own inner voice.

More than anything, I have an intense desire to share what I have learned with those who seek the same truth—how to live their very best life, one of honesty, freedom, authenticity, choice, and ultimately health and longevity. The French style of eating—sitting down with delight and savoring every bite with discretion, moderation, and passion—is the answer. ✥

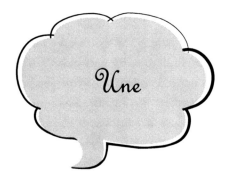

Une

Le Poids Naturel
Your Natural Weight

You have to leave the city of your comfort and go into the wilderness of your intuition. What you will discover will be wonderful. What you will discover is yourself.

—Alan Alda

"ON EST INDIVIDUALISTE!" boasts the French woman. Her beauty is expressed and exhibited in many packages, and the differences are appealing, even desirable. The French woman is perhaps a short, "bohemian" redhead with freckles and lovely curls, a tall, voluptuous blonde strolling l'avenue Montaigne, or a sixty-five-year-old grandmother who presents herself *au natural.* Each woman is considered beautiful in her own right.

And whether the French woman is a single, career-minded Parisian or a mother living in a rural village far from the city, she strives to embrace the essence of a meaningful life. She cannot be defined in a fashion magazine. She is her own woman.

By contrast, many Americans tend to relate beauty to the latest movie star or cultural icon, imitating a hairstyle, clothing, perhaps even their idol's workout regimen.

So here is the first secret we can learn from the French woman: Embracing your individuality and beauty while at the same time accepting your body at its natural weight will you get back to the business of living and create room for endless joy, health, and longevity. It's exactly that joy that creates radiance regardless of your age or shape. It's the *je ne sais quoi* we find so alluring in the French woman.

Back to the French girl, who is absolutely content at her natural weight, no matter what her shape or size: There's no doubt that she does have a tendency to be thin—and there *is* pressure in France to be thin, if only to fit into the clothes. In the boutiques where I shopped I don't think I saw a garment that was above a size 10.

NATURAL WEIGHT IS . . .

↣ The weight that results from healthy eating and regular exercise.

↣ The weight that individuals making reasonable changes in their diet and exercise patterns can seek and maintain over a period of time.

↣ The weight at which one is relatively free of health problems.

The difference is that the French woman is not preoccupied with diet and exercise. This American obsession has no place in her world. She is much too involved in living and learning, and in enjoying such undemanding and reliably rewarding pleasures as food and sex, to count calories.

In France, weight management is a private matter, to be handled quietly by simply modifying the way a woman eats and by walking a little faster in her high heels. French women (and their men!) embrace a little flesh—a hard body is not at all what they're after.

Why We Don't Accept Our Natural Weight

Who decides what is the perfect weight or body shape for you? How do you *know* that you should weigh 120 pounds, that your hips are too wide or your breasts too small? If your answer is that your mother or your husband told you so, then let's ask the question another way: Who told *them* that's the perfect weight or body?

To a large degree, the answer is that our culture (including our friends, family, schools, communities) sends us these messages. Think about how many of your ideas come from your parents, teachers, co-workers, boyfriends, husbands, friends, and sisters. After such reflection, many of us realize that those closest to us have an enormous influence on our beliefs and standards.

But this is normal, you may say, and has happened throughout human history. The difference is that in this country we have allowed this influence to penetrate into our very ideas of ourselves.

And by what mechanism has the culture imposed its authority on you? Could it be simply that we are all victims of the American media?

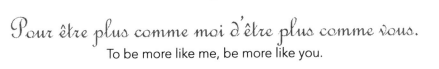

Pour être plus comme moi d'être plus comme vous.
To be more like me, be more like you.

A study reported in the journal *Sex Roles* has found that pictures of female models in magazines can exert a powerful influence on a woman's feelings about her own body. Researchers from the University of Missouri–Columbia (UM) measured how a group of women felt about themselves after viewing models in magazine ads for one to three minutes. In all cases, the women, *regardless of their weight and size*, reported a drop in their level of satisfaction with their bodies.* "Surprisingly, we found that weight was not a factor. Viewing these pictures was just bad for everyone," said UM's Laurie Mintz. "It had been thought that women who are heavier feel worse than a thinner woman after viewing pictures of the thin ideal in the mass media. The study results do not support that theory."

Right now today, could you make an unconditional relationship with yourself? Just at the height you are, the weight you are, the amount of intelligence that you have, the burden of pain that you have?
—Pema Chodron, "Start Where You Are"

The study suggests that reducing the acceptance of mass media images of women and trying to stop the social comparison process is important for helping all women. "Most women do not go to a counselor for advice; they look to *Seventeen* or *Glamour* magazine instead," Mintz said. "These unrealistic images of women, which are often airbrushed or partially computer generated have a detrimental impact on women and how they feel about themselves."

How do women feel? Based on my work as a nutritionist, I say they suffer from low self-esteem, body image distortions, and unrealistic expectations. Because our bodies can't possibly resemble the ideals set up by the media, our children and young adults learn early on to dismiss their individuality and to embrace standards that are distorted and impossible to attain.

The situation could not be more different for the women of France, who are nurtured and encouraged to embrace their individuality and eccentricity. French women also know that being a little shorter or taller or a little more heavily built can be healthy and attractive.

To paraphrase the words of Wendy Oliver Pyatt, M.D, in her book *Fed Up!* we should be ashamed that as parents, teachers, and adults we have fallen into the clutches of the media and of a culture that created and admired a doll named Barbie, who, if she were a real woman, would have to walk on all fours because she's too top-heavy and otherwise emaciated to stand upright.

What Influences Our Natural Weight?

Not all of us struggle to manage our weight—a situation that can be attributed primarily to our individual genetic differences. Genetic makeup determines an individual's susceptibility to obesity when she is exposed to an unfavorable environment, such as low-quality processed foods and/or a sedentary lifestyle, as well as her ability to respond to diet and exercise.

Many studies that have shown that a tendency to be obese is genetic have examined the interactions of a person's genes and lifestyle as obesity develops. The studies have identified certain DNA sequence variations called single nucleotide polymorphisms (SNPs) that respond to diet and exercise. Some SNPs make some people more sensitive to the amount of fat in the diet, while others make some people more resistant to exercise-induced weight loss.*

And some people suffer from self-inflicted metabolic problems, ones they bring on themselves through dieting. Restricting calories lowers your metabolism because when your body is deprived of calories it becomes more efficient, requiring fewer calories to perform the daily functions that are necessary for survival. And over-restriction of calorie intake is typically linked to subsequent periods of over-eating, or bingeing.*

I once asked a math professor friend just what he liked about his subject. He said, "That's easy. I love math because there's only one right answer."

And I said, "That's exactly why I don't like math!"

In weight management there is no one answer that fits everyone, no one simple, universal answer to be found on the scale or in a formula as simple as: calories in − calories out = ideal body weight.

It's all about you!

Conveniently enough, there is one number that is specific and important to you—your basal metabolic rate. The BMR is a number that confirms your uniqueness. Sure, you have a lot in common with other people, but at the foundation you are one of a kind: Your age, height, gender, and current weight all determine how many calories it takes to maintain your body at rest, even when you're sleeping. That number of calories is your BMR.

If you have noticed that every year it becomes harder to eat whatever you want and stay slim, you know that your BMR decreases as you age. What you may not understand is that depriving yourself of food in the hope of losing weight also decreases your BMR. One study* showed that the BMR can drop by about 30 percent when calories are abruptly and seriously reduced, and another* showed that low-calorie weight-loss diets can cause drops in BMR of up to 20 percent.

After twenty years of age, the typical person's BMR reduces by 2 percent every decade. The good news is that as your body's ability to burn energy gradually slows down with age, regular exercise in the form of everyday movement can increase your BMR and improve your health and fitness.

The Harris Benedict equation, laid out below for both women and men, is a calorie formula using the factors of height, weight, age, and gender to determine basal metabolic rate. The inclusion of all of these factors makes this equation more accurate than determining calorie needs based on total body weight alone. The only variable it does not take into consideration is lean body mass.

This equation will be very accurate in all but the extremely muscular (in that case, it will underestimate caloric needs) and the extremely overweight (for these people, it will overestimate caloric needs). Here are the equations for women and for men:

Femmes: 661 + (4.38 x weight in pounds) + (4.38 x height in inches) – (4.7 x age) = BMR

Hommes: 67 + (6.24 x weight in pounds) + (12.7 x height in inches) – (6.9 x age) = BMR

Let's do the equation for a forty-year-old man who is 6 feet tall (72 inches) and weighs 175 pounds:

67 + (6.24 x 175) + (12.7 x 72) – (6.9 x 40) = BMR
67 + 1,092 + 914.4 – 276 = 1,797.40

The man in our example utilizes 1,797.4 calories at rest.

To determine additional calories you consume through activity, you need to use a multiplier. To determine, based on your basal metabolism and activity level, the total number of calories you require each day to stay at your present weight, multiply your BMR by the one of the following numbers, depending on your activity level. The resulting number is known as your Total Daily Energy Expenditure (TDEE).

Sedentary	x 1.15
Light activity (normal, everyday activities)	x 1.3
Moderately active (exercise 3 to 4 times a week)	x 1.4
Very active (exercise more than 4 times a week)	x 1.6
Extremely active (exercise 6 to 7 times a week)	x 1.8

If the man in our example is a very active person, we would multiply 1,797.4 (his BMR) by 1.6 (very active) and get 2,875.84 as the total calories he utilizes each day. This means that on a daily basis, his weight will not change if he eats approximately 2,875.84 calories each day and continues to exercise.

As you can see, men and women differ greatly in these calculations: A man's BMR is typically higher than a woman's. Because of their genetic makeup men have more muscle than women, and consequently their metabolisms are higher because lean muscle utilizes more calories than fat. Men's bodies have 3 percent essential body fat, while women's have 12 percent; therefore, men, with their higher proportion of muscle, hold a significant advantage in caloric expenditure.

Weight Regulation 101

We know that 3,500 calories equal one pound. Taking into account that you should never eat less than 1,000 calories a day, never skip meals, and never over-exercise, a numbers approach to weight management can be calculated in the following manner, keeping in mind that numbers alone are not the whole equation:

To lose 1 pound a week (3,500 calories), reduce your daily caloric intake by 500 (7 x 500 = 3,500). The same goes for gaining weight—but in reverse. Increasing caloric intake by 500 calories a day over your total daily energy expenditure for seven days will result in a one-pound weight gain.

The man in the previous example expends 2,875.84 a day, and let's say that his weight remains stable because he eats roughly that many calories daily. If he reduces his daily caloric intake by 500 (to 2,375.84), he will safely lose one pound per week. And by the way, losing one pound a week is a realistic, safe, and sustainable approach to weight management. Again, no quick fix or hocus-pocus.

In my experience working with a diverse group of clients, I have learned that understanding the biological math helps weight management become less emotional and more scientific. Because it "is what it is," many individuals who learn these basic metabolic facts are able to navigate their weight management much as they do different aspects of their lives, such as their business careers or personal finances.

When you operate a business, you work within a profit-and-loss structure. Spend too much and your business is in the red. Spend too much over a long period of time and you're out of business.

Eat too much for a week or so and you become slightly overweight. Eat too much over a long period of time and you become obese. If you are able to create this connection between weight management and the other important areas of your life, you will not "overspend" in terms of the amount you eat. As my client John told me, he's fine with the numbers and works within the guidelines, keeping his weight in check, and on any given day he has never "left money on the table."

French Women Just Won't Get Fat

I can assure you that the French are not swapping stories about their BMR—if they even know what it is. Instead, on an intrinsic level they learn, from childhood on, how to regulate their weight through simple steps such as eating when they are hungry, eating slowly enough to know when they are almost full, and dining in a state of relaxation and thus heightened assimilation. And if indeed their clothes feel a bit tight, they will automatically adjust their servings until things are zipping up nicely again.

It's not so much that French women *don't* get fat—it's more that they refuse to. They just *won't* get fat.

Cornell University researchers agree that the French use internal cues—such as no longer feeling hungry—to stop eating. Americans, on the other hand, tend to use external cues—their plate is clean, they have finished their beverage, or the TV show they're watching is over.

"Furthermore, we have found that the heavier a person is—French or American—the more they rely on external cues to tell them to stop eating and the less they rely on whether they felt full," said Cornell's Brian Wansink, co-author of a study that analyzes questionnaires from Parisians and Chicagoans about how they decide when to stop eating.*

"Over-relying on external cues to stop eating a meal may prove useful in offering a partial explanation of why body mass index varies across people and potentially across cultures," said co-author Collin Payne, a Cornell postdoctoral researcher. "Relying on internal cues for meal cessation, rather than on external cues, may improve eating patterns in the long term."

I've shared the BMR formula with you not so that you will become obsessed with the numbers. I've laid out this simple reasoning to help you make sense of the differences that account for our individuality, differences that include height, weight, gender, and age and that require individually tailored eating plans rather than boilerplate regimens.

Here's an example of what happens in my household because I have this information: When I prepare salmon for dinner, I serve my husband a larger piece than myself. He's more than double my weight, his gender gives him an edge because his body has a greater proportion of lean muscle mass, and he's a lot taller than me. Because of these physical characteristics, his body requires more food than mine. So rather than try to eat as much as he does or ask why life is so unfair, I accept the physiology and be sure that I throw a few extra servings his way so that I have room for dessert. The joke in our house is that "a man of his stature" just needs more food!

There is no need to count calories or step on the scale. Just as with the household budget, after a couple of bounced checks you get a feel for things and know when you're close to overspending, even if you don't scrutinize your cash flow on a daily basis.

Intuitive eating will eventually take over the BMR formula in your mind, but until such time you will have a scientific way to help in defining your personal boundaries. My advice—spend all of your calories every day on the most delectable dishes available. Bon appétit!

Being Underweight Is Bad for Your Health

Contrary to the old adage "You can never be too rich or too thin," being overly skinny carries its own health risks. Being underweight is defined as having a body mass index (BMI) below 18.5. For example, someone who is 5 feet 5 inches tall and weighs 110 pounds would have a BMI of 18.3, which is considered underweight.

Juliette couldn't make peace with her normal weight. "When I was in the hospital I was at my perfect weight—ten pounds thinner," she bragged.

I reminded her, "You were *in the hospital*, sick, weak, and struggling to recover—and, by the way, *skeletal!*"

"Yea, I know, I was *so* thin." She went on, "The bar has been set, and that's my goal!"

Thank you, Juliette, for providing a perfect example of the unrealistic and absurd expectations of dieting and distorted body image.

Many of my clients complain that the last five pounds are very difficult to lose. My theory is that, in the divine wisdom of the creator, our body holds on to these few pounds to ensure our safety when we do fall ill, to allow our bodies the energy required to fight the illness and recover safely.

Don't Weaken Your Immune System!

When a person's weight drops critically low, it's harder for the body to absorb nutrients. According to an article in *Today's Dietitian*, reduced absorption of amino acids, vitamins, and minerals can lead to a variety of harmful conditions.* For example, when calcium isn't consumed and absorbed in proper amounts, a person's risk for osteoporosis (weak, fragile bones) increases, while lack of iron commonly leads to anemia (iron deficiency). Other conditions related to poor nutrient absorption include digestive concerns, amenorrhea (loss of a woman's menstrual cycle), and difficulty with pregnancy.

HOW TO CALCULATE YOUR BMI

Body mass index calculation requires only two measurements: height and weight.

BMI = weight (pounds) ÷ height (inches) squared x 703

Let's do the calculation for a 120-pound woman who is 5 feet 5 inches tall.

1. Calculate the number of inches.
   5 x 12 = 60 + 5 = 65 inches

2. Calculate the number of inches squared (multiply the number of inches by the same number).
   65 x 65 = 4,225

3. Divide the weight in pounds by the height in inches squared.
   120 ÷ 4,225 = 0.0284

4. Multiply that answer by 703.
   0.0284 x 703 = 19.97

The result: a BMI of 19.97 (normal).

BMI WEIGHT STATUS CATEGORIES

BMI	Weight Status
Below 18.5	Underweight
18.5–24.9	Normal
25–29.9	Overweight
30 + above	Obese

For an online BMI calculator, visit whathealth.com/bmi/forumula.html.

Gravely underweight individuals have poor physical stamina and a weak immune system, opening them to a risk of infection. Clinical dietitian Elena Blanco-Schumacher explains that the 8 to 9 percent of America's population who are considered underweight generally carry reduced body mass, a characteristic that increases risk for infections.

Underweight individuals are also likely to consume too little protein, fat, and other nutrients, such as antioxidants, that help maintain a strong, working immune system. When underweight individuals develop infections or disease, their bodies are less able to fight them and the conditions may continue and worsen.

Let's expand our definition of beauty and reject cultural values that make perfectly fine (in fact, often exquisite) people feel overweight and ugly. By taking a realistic look at your genetic background, your age and hormonal status, as well as your BMR, you can find your natural weight.

If you are a serial dieter, it is time to accept the body you own. If you have given up altogether and resigned yourself to a life of obesity, think again! Reject the unnatural cultural values and counterproductive dieting that have kept you overweight. Throw off the self-imposed chains that bind you! Free yourself to let your body naturally shed its excess weight if you are overweight, and discover your own natural beauty. Live the life you deserve.

PRACTICING YOUR FRENCH

This week:

1. Pursue a diet of healthy ideas—read, write, explore, solve. Resist mental stagnation with a sense of discovery and adventure.
2. Replace the abandon of overeating by finding opportunities for art and beauty in the smallest and most basic chores.
3. Gather the important women in your life in a book group that focuses on breaking the cycle of preoccupation with food, preventing it from being handed down to another generation of women. Begin with Wendy Oliver-Pyatt's book *Fed-Up!* and help end the tyranny of unrealistic and dangerous cultural stereotypes.

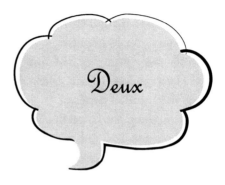

Deux

Pas de Résistance
No Resistance

Ce que vous résistez persiste:
That which you resist persists.

—*Unknown*

THANK YOU VERY MUCH, Isaac Newton, for your third law of motion, which describes the relationship between the forces acting on a body and that body's motion. The simple truth is that the more you push something away, the more it comes back, now or later—in relation to eating, mostly in the form of a craving for *pain au chocolat*. Never dieting is the second secret of the French woman.

When I began practicing nutrition my first surprise was realizing that, in order to be effective, I might need a degree in psychology along with credentials in nutrition. It turns out that, more often than not, issues revolving around food are more emotional and subjective than scientific and practical.

Having struggled through biology, I found this quite disheartening. It seemed that very few of my clients wanted to talk about or even cared about the health benefits of a sweet potato. No matter the size, shape, or gender of the individual, their questions always circled back to diet and weight loss.

Another surprise was that most people wanted to be told what to eat and were quite uncomfortable when I wouldn't give them a list of do's and don'ts. They wanted the dogma of a diet plan.

I'll give you an example. A wonderful young female executive whom I will call Marcelle came to my office for an initial consultation. She was of average size and above-average intelligence. Marcelle held a prestigious position and seemed very much in control of her life.

I consider my first meeting with a client an intake session in which I learn about the person's medical history and food preferences. Marcelle and I had an informative and comfortable first session, and I felt I had a good handle on a plan that I would present to her as we proceeded.

We scheduled our next session, and as Marcelle stood up to leave, she asked, "What should I have for lunch today?"

I answered, "What are you in the mood for? There's a great café across the street that serves the most wonderful sandwiches." As I continued to elaborate on the freshness of the food and the cleanliness of the place, she fell back into the chair, weeping.

Dumbfounded, I grabbed a tissue for her and asked what I could do to help. Between sobs she said, "I haven't eaten bread in two years . . . I want it, it sounds delicious, but I'm so afraid of carbs—I'll gain weight."

Resistance to a piece of bread, a simple item made of flour and water, had reduced an otherwise intelligent woman to tears and left her craving the most basic of foods. Not to mention that after all of her deprivation she had not reached her desired weight.

Honestly, can you imagine any self-respecting French woman giving up her morning croissant *for two years?* The French deny themselves very little when it comes to food. They avoid anything that requires too much effort for too little pleasure, and they know that denial is not healthy (and that balance is essential).

And since French women are individuals, they don't follow mass movements, particularly when it comes to food. French women do not diet.

If Marcelle had been expecting a diet, she was in the wrong place. My goal as a nutritionist is to empower an individual to live her very best and most pleasurable life through an approach to eating that is based on whole foods and that supports health.

This goal can be achieved only by stripping away outside influences, beginning with the distraction of diets, and getting back in touch with one's own desires, preferences, palate, heritage, genetics, traditions, lifestyle, and uniqueness. Until such time as this shift occurs, our emotional and physical hungers will remain bottomless and insatiable.

My Definition of "Diet": Not Having a Mind of Your Own

Dieting is the ultimate betrayal. There is no more efficient way to lose touch with yourself and your body's cues than to restrict your eating. Dieting is the best way to assure that that you will re-gain any weight you lose, plus some.

Americans are obsessed with dieting, whether it's trying to follow some expert's scheme or just restricting their calories. I'm not sure how we got into this fine mess, but it's time to acknowledge that it is not our body that betrays us; it is we who betray our body.

I was talking and stretching with Felice, my yoga instructor, after a recent session. Felice was excited about attending a yoga conference out of town and wanted to be at her best since she would be meeting and working with her peers and reuniting with old friends. She is an enlightened sort of person, so it surprised me when she mentioned that she planned to skip dinner for a few nights in preparation for the event. She wanted to drop a few pounds before the conference.

We have a wonderful and close relationship, so I said, "Felice, let me ask you a question—are you hungry at dinner time?"

She answered, "Yeah, but I'll ignore it."

I said, "Really? You'll *ignore* it?"

"Yeah, I can do that for a couple nights. I have a goal," she replied in a self-righteous sort of way.

"Wow," I said, "that's amazing. When you need to use the toilet, do you ignore that, too?"

She looked stunned.

I repeated myself more graphically this time, "So when you have bodily urges like peeing, do you just hold it in?"

"Of course not," she laughed.

"Or better yet," I asked, "when you don't have the urge to pee, do you try to force it anyway?"

"I get it, I get it—you made your point," she said thoughtfully.

Even the most enlightened of us succumb to the madness of dieting. For me, it was a way to control my universe, or so I thought. My thinking was that I may not be able to control the events around me, but I certainly can control what I eat.

This type of thinking is really a slippery slope, and I was fortunate not to slide any further along it than I did. I fell into the category of disordered eating. Many are less fortunate and end up with severe and life-threatening eating disorders such as anorexia and bulimia.

DISORDERED EATING OR EATING DISORDER?

The many types of "disordered" (irregular) eating habits that do not warrant diagnosis as an eating disorder include excluding whole food groups (such as all fats or all carbohydrates), eating only at particular times of day, eating only specific foods, eating only foods of a particular color, eating only foods with a specific texture, and not eating certain foods together.

Sometimes these habits form in childhood in a person who's labeled a "picky eater." People can also use such patterns as part of a quest to control weight or as coping mechanisms against emotional stress, as in my case.

Psychiatrists also use "disordered eating" as a category for eating patterns that meet some but not all of the criteria for an eating disorder like anorexia or bulimia. For example, a girl who fits all of the criteria for anorexia but remains within a normal weight range or continues to have menstrual periods may be diagnosed as having disordered eating. Similarly, someone who binge-eats and purges occasionally but not frequently enough to be diagnosed as bulimic is usually described as exhibiting disordered eating.

And it can all start with a diet. It's like putting your hand in a flame and thinking you won't get burned. Trust me—you always get burned when you diet. You always lose touch with yourself. You always feel as though your nose is pressed against a window and those on the other side are living fully and enjoying what you are not. This is no way to live. Stop the madness.

Never before have we had greater access to facts, figures, comparisons, and rich data when it comes to weight management. Statistics abound concerning calories, fat grams, carbohydrates, BMI, belly fat—you name it, we've heard about it on the *Today* show or the nightly news and read about it on the Web and in every magazine ever printed and in any number of bestselling books.

There's even an application on the iPhone that allows you to log every morsel you consume, every calorie you burn. Famous people endorse diet centers, lose the weight, and gain it back just in time to star in their own reality show and give it another try.

When you choose a diet over intuitive eating
you opt for one of two likely outcomes:

→ Diet, lose the weight, and gain it back—plus some.

→ Diet, lose the weight, and spend the rest of your life
in deprivation for fear of regaining the pounds.

Speaking of reality shows, they got it right when they named *The Biggest Loser*. The show publicly humiliates obese individuals who lose hundreds of pounds in a controlled environment on camera—only to gain the weight back in the real world and then return to the show.

Of course they gain it back! Who can exercise five hours a day in the real world—who *wants* to? These shows are successful; their ratings are high, and they produce outstanding profits, but what do they accomplish aside from providing some indecorous "entertainment" while endorsing a destructive dieting mentality? When a show like this comes on, pick up the remote control or, better yet, walk to the TV set and turn it off. Do not allow this propaganda, disguised as a television program, to become your reality.

Keep in mind that, even though the media has extensive and unprecedented access to authorities on weight management, and despite all the weight-loss products and low-this and reduced-that offerings on the supermarket shelves, obesity rates in America are at an all-time high. Americans are having no success managing their weight. What gives? I'll tell you what gives . . .

We're Drowning in Information and Thirsty for Wisdom

Wisdom is the knowledge of what is true or right coupled with judgment, discernment, and insight. How can we expect to have insight when we are constantly looking outside ourselves for the answers and inadvertently absorbing information that often has nothing to do with our lives?

Weight management is an inside job. Mother Nature didn't pull a dirty trick on us in providing such a bounty of wonderful things to eat. We just stopped listening to her.

A year or so ago I received a call from one of my dearest friends, Suzette, who was spending the year living in another state. She couldn't wait to tell me her news. "Carol, I've lost so much weight! The pounds are falling off—I've lost more than thirty-five so far!" she sang.

I love Suzette, and for a brief moment I was right there with her in wonderland. But, alas, I have far too much experience with this fairy tale. I quickly sprang back to reality, and I have to confess that my mind wandered a bit as she shared her secret.

"It's low-glycemic and, you see, it was never my fault—I'm an addict, a sugar and carb addict. Now I have the answer."

Suzette and I have discussed this low-glycemic notion in the past, and I agree that each and every one of us would benefit by discovering our own "tipping point"—the point at which sugar triggers our appetite and becomes something resembling a runaway train.

My weakness is and always has been sweets. I'll never overdose on potato chips or fatty foods, but sweets—that's another story altogether. So I have learned to develop a sixth sense, one that requires staying present when I enjoy treats.

For me it's like driving on a treacherous road in an ice storm—I keep two hands on the wheel and admit no distractions. That way I see it coming—the next turn, a patch of ice, whatever. The point is that I am in the driver's seat. I decide how to take the turns.

Most of the time I'm happy with one cookie—maybe one and a half—rather than a dozen. The trick is to remember that there is always another treat in your future.

When you give up the dieting mentality, you can take a deep breath, relax, and know that, just as there was today, there will be something special offered tomorrow. There is no need to eat every last cookie or donut, meanwhile promising a fresh start on Monday, or after the vacation, or after the full moon, or whatever deal you make with yourself.

Nine out of ten times this method is effective, but because we are human and because we have spent so many years eating for reasons other than hunger, a slip-up is to be expected every now and then. Even after several years of practicing what I'm preaching here, when I am stressed there is a greater chance that one cookie will lead to two and the thought of three.

But notice I said *thought*. I will stop before the train leaves the station because, to mix a few metaphors, I am awake at the plate and I know my tipping point. This is the wisdom I speak of: your very own wisdom, not a program, a workshop, a diet—you name the plan: Skinny Bitch, Zone, Atkins, South Beach—or an "addiction."

It's true that the French deny themselves very little when it comes to food. But they also eat very little of it: a piece of dark chocolate after a meal, as opposed to a large piece (or two) of cake. They know that denial isn't healthy but that indulgence has to be moderated.

The French also have an automatic habit of exercising caution after a period of excess. Eating more today makes them more careful tomorrow. Rather than diet, they would rather regularly trade off a large meal or two with a few lighter ones.

What happened to Suzette, you ask? You already know because you've seen this movie many times, but I'll tell you anyway. She came back into town and couldn't wait to meet me and show off her new figure and, yes, she looked wonderful. We met with our husbands for brunch. She chose the place so she could stay on plan.

As I watched her picking crumbs from the bread basket, I knew she was at the end of the road with this low-glycemic scheme. She ordered the omelet with this and that left out, on the side and upside down, while my husband and I shared the crab crepes and apple streusel pancakes. She tapped her fork in the streusel topping from my plate and, with her fork to her mouth as if the utensil were a gun loaded with one bullet in a game of Russian roulette, she tasted the syrupy topping.

Week by week, pound by pound, Suzette put the weight back on, until one day she called me from out of town once more and cried, "I'm fat!"

A year later, Suzette and I had lunch again, and again she named the place. You see, she'd been out of town, following a trip on a runaway train and into her routine again, working with the nutritionist who'd put her on the glycemic thing last year. "Today it's been one week that I'm back on plan," she announced. "And I feel great."

Here we sit, more than a year later, she with her vegetables and me with whatever I want—only she's heavier and I'm thinner. As I dropped her off at her place, I wondered if she saw the irony in our choices and outcomes. And as I thought about it on the drive home, I understood that she just doesn't know what else to do . . . this is how it's done.

Dieting is what we've been taught. Even though it's the dieting that isn't effective, Suzette is willing to accept the blame: She did it wrong, she doesn't have willpower, she's a carb and sugar addict. She needs a do-over, a fresh start.

If you ask me, she's addicted to fresh starts and a clean slate more than to carbs and sugar. Like so many other dieters, she doesn't trust herself and has tuned out her inner voice and innate wisdom.

Feel Free to Be Your Unique Self

"Where do you want to go for lunch?" Suzette asked, as she pulled up in her shiny new car to greet me another year later. The car was new, the question was not. "Sushi?" she threw out.

"No, I'm not in the mood today," I said, surprising myself with a rather awkward, rapid response. Generally, I let Suzette decide since often she is eliminating something—carbs, sugar, maybe meat. Even though I don't approve of her dieting and even more abhor the voluntary confinement her dieting conviction creates, I do respect the process and the time that unraveling this thinking requires.

But for whatever reason, on this day I jumped in with, "How about the Turkish place? We can split what we ordered last time." Her eyes sparkled for a moment before her typical fear overshadowed her enthusiasm. Quite unconsciously, I determined that this was the right decision.

Along the way to the Turkish restaurant, we passed the French bakery, where I stopped to grab a closer look at the plate of a sidewalk diner and then gaze into the café for a review of the day's offerings in the pastry case. I might need to save a bit of room, I decided silently.

Suzette was drooling, so I asked if she would rather eat here, at the French café.

"No, I'll be bad," she said in the voice of a five-year-old.

"OK, onward to the Turkish place," I said.

We got seated and were ready to order. Suzette asked our server about the salad and the chicken kabob.

I quickly interrupted. "Last time we were here we split the *ispanakli pide*, the spinach, feta, and tomato pastry that comes with a salad—remember?"

"Oh yeah, oh yeah—I guess I was thinking of the time before," she mumbled. I knew that Suzette preferred the savory pastry. I sat patiently, though I was keenly aware of her ritual. She was moralizing and sanctioning the lean kabob, the perfect

CHOCOLAT

The film *Chocolat* (2000) pits sensual pleasure against disciplined self-denial, and the most tempting of all sweets is the key weapon in the battle. It's 1959 and a mysterious woman named Vianne (Juliette Binoche) moves with her daughter to a small French village.

Shortly after Lent begins, Vianne opens a confectionary shop across from the church. The townspeople are supposed to abstain from worldly pleasures, but Vianne tempts them with delicious chocolate creations, offering the right concoction to break down each customer's resistance.

With every passing day, more of Vianne's neighbors succumb to her sinful treats, but the Comte de Reynaud (Alfred Molina), the town's mayor, is not amused; he wants Vianne run out of town before she leads the populace into a deeper level of temptation. Instead, with the help of a handsome Irish Gypsy named Roux (Johnny Depp), Vianne plans a Grand Festival of Chocolate, to be held on Easter Sunday.

The church stands for tradition, for the way things have always been, and, especially during Lent, for self-restraint and sacrifice. The mayor leans on the young parish priest, just five weeks on the job, to reinforce such values from the pulpit. Père Henri (Hugh O'Conor) dutifully preaches sermons about the dangers of temptation, the threat to morality posed by outsiders, even the evils of chocolate.

Until Easter morning, when Père Henri tells his parishioners he doesn't want to talk about Jesus's divinity. He is more interested in what we can learn from his life on earth: "I'd rather talk about his humanity . . . His kindness, his tolerance . . . We can't go around . . . measuring our goodness by what we don't do. By what we deny ourselves, what we resist, and who we exclude . . . We've got to measure goodness by what we embrace."

The newcomer priest provides the perfect message for our culture of crazy dieting: Witness the insanity that surrounds you! Embrace your life and eat up every sweet morsel of goodness. Above all, be kind and tolerant not only to others, but first, and above all, to yourself.

protein-dominant meal—she's a carb *addict*, after all. Somewhere out of pure instinct I knew it was now or never. I ordered the pastry.

"I've written about you in my book," I revealed.

"Really?" she replied inquisitively, a tinge of fear in her voice.

"Yup, I wrote about our last couple of lunches."

"*Hmmmm,*" she mumbled under her breath, her mind clearly in express-playback mode. Afraid of disclosing too much, and at the same time knowing that I was on the right track, I dropped the subject for a few moments in order to gain a little perspective and a dose of bravado.

We were back to catching up and sharing observations about current events when the meal arrived. I observed Suzette's expression illuminate in delight! The pastry was nestled within an artful mound of shredded carrots, beets, and mixed greens. It was lovely to look at, and the aroma was heavenly. We savored the Turkish specialty, and as was only natural, somewhere in between delectable bites, I sensed the wall that stood between her diet and my indulgence collapsing. Suzette was being drawn blissfully toward the light.

I took full advantage of the occasion, elaborating on my theories regarding the French and the freedom to be one's unique self. Suzette was there—*finally*. I held back my own tears as I watched Suzette's lower lip quiver. An eyewitness to the instantaneous relaxation of her body as she surrendered to a life of freedom, choice, and authenticity, I remembered my own journey. There have been a handful of times in my practice when I have known the importance of the work that I am engaged in. This was certainly one of those times.

Move Up to the Palace

When a woman refuses to move the mental parameters of a diet, her life becomes limited and small.

I am reminded of the fable about a princess kidnapped at a young age and taken to live as a pauper among fishmongers. Over time she adopted the fishmongers' lifestyle. Years later her royal parents discovered her whereabouts and brought her back to her room in the palace. There she found a large, soft bed, clean linens, flowers, exotic fruit, incense, and elegant clothing, and she was serenaded by chamber music played outside her door.

That night the princess lay awake, tossing and turning. "Let me out of here," she beseeched her attendants. "I can't stand the smell, and this place feels weird."

The princess had grown so used to the smell of fish and a lifestyle of deprivation that a more refined atmosphere seemed foreign and repulsive to her. Many of us have become accustomed to foods that taste like paper and have forgotten our royal heritage. We need to be reminded to dine like kings and queens rather than peasants. We also have become too accustomed to a coarse and smelly world. We have accepted lack, loss, and limitation in the form of a diet as the norm. But dieting and fake foods do not befit the life we were born to live.

DOCUMENT THE DOGMA

Make a list of all the diets you've tried, starting with the very
first one. Note how long each diet lasted, and how you felt when
you started and then again when you finished. Did you lose weight? Did
you keep the weight off? If so, for what period of time?
Record the results to see what all that deprivation got you.

Like the princess, when wonderful things like self-indulgence and freedom come along, we may feel uncomfortable and out of place and subconsciously resist those pleasurable conditions, or even sabotage our ability to accept them.

In the same way, my dear friend Suzette stands witness to my all-inclusive, gratifying dining experiences and a lifestyle of free choice, yet she ascribes my leaner physique to a stroke of luck—I must have a faster metabolism and she must have a flaw in her metabolic makeup. Not dieting really feels weird to Suzette. But there is nothing weird about health, fitness, and longevity.

It's deprivation, obesity, the victim mentality, and failure that should feel weird to us because they do not match our nature or our purpose. Yet we put up with them and keep recreating them simply because they are familiar.

Right now, take some time to consider if you are settling for fishmonger conditions and denying yourself your rightful room in the palace. If so, take a breath and try to remember who you really are and what you truly deserve.

There's another wise woman we tend to tune out. She's 151 feet tall, holds a book and a torch on high, and stands at the entrance to New York Harbor. *La Liberté Eclairant le Monde* (*Liberty Enlightening the World*) was a gift of friendship from the people of France to the United States to commemorate the 100th anniversary of American independence. Her more familiar American name is *The Statue of Liberty*. Smaller versions of the statue also stand in two places in Paris: the Île des Cygnes (Swan Island) in the River Seine and the Luxembourg Gardens. They are all symbols of friendship, freedom, and peace between the United States and France.

Let them be a reminder that liberty is the condition of being free from restriction or control—the right and power to act, believe, and express yourself in a manner of your choosing. What a gift indeed! *Merci beaucoup!*

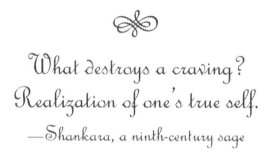

What destroys a craving?
Realization of one's true self.
—Shankara, a ninth-century sage

The Key to Weight Management: Self-Affirmation

My husband, John, is a twin, a ten-pound-heavier version of his otherwise identical brother. When I met John's twin I expected to not only see but also *feel* similarities between the two. To my surprise, even though they are identical physically—notwithstanding the ten-pound variance—they are very different individuals. John's brother is more deliberate and analytical, and my husband is more social and communicative. And unlike his brother, my husband is very emotionally driven to impulsive acts, such as eating when he's stressed.

A few years ago, researchers at Charles University, in the Czech Republic, did a study of weight loss and metabolic efficiency in twins in order to assess how much our genes contribute to our body's ability to lose weight. The study found that the degree of metabolic efficiency within pairs of twins is very similar.* In other words, my husband and his brother may be different in certain personality traits, but their metabolisms burn calories at the same rate.

So the extra ten pounds that my husband carries is simply due to the fact that *he eats more than his twin*. John's impulsive eating is what makes him ten pounds heavier than his genetic counterpart.

A truly successful weight-management approach is one that deals with an individual's self-image as well as the underlying emotional needs that cause overeating. Often overeating stems from a sense of feeling emotionally undernourished; in such cases, there is a misguided attempt to use food to replace soul satisfaction. People can put on weight as a result of feelings of insecurity or anxiety or depression or any of a long list of emotional ills. The point is that it is not possible to take off the pounds without dealing with the mind-set.

In the words of Alan Cohen, my longtime guru and the author of inspirational books in the fields of personal growth, inspiration, holistic health, human relations, and work and life balance:

> If you can rediscover the inner beauty with which you were created, you will make a major stride toward successful weight loss or any other avenue of self-improvement. Ultimately, we heal only by getting to know and love the self we are already in. The way out is in. The path to freedom is to return to your source. At your center lives a being so radiant and magnificent that upon beholding it you will lovingly laugh at the notion of trying to improve what God made whole. Then you are free to enjoy what you are. Give up your efforts to become perfect by accepting the perfection in which you were created.

PRACTICING YOUR FRENCH

This week:

1. Toss your diet books and replace them with French cookbooks.
2. Tune out media influences. Don't read diet ads, and don't watch television commercials that promote dieting.

Trois

La Qualité
Quality

It's a funny thing about life; if you accept anything but the very best, you will get it.

— W. Somerset Maugham

IN THE FRENCH WAY of life, quality is everything—our book's third secret. When it comes to food, quality means real, fresh, locally produced, and mindfully prepared. No matter what their income level, the French know that you get what you pay for. They accept only the very best their budget will permit. This reverence and respect for food also means that there is little waste; shopping is accomplished with mindfulness, one meal at a time, with emphasis on a few simple, fresh ingredients. Whether they are eating at home or dining out, our French friends choose the highest-quality foods available.

Carolyn's Story

"I grew up in the suburbs of Chicago amid mega strip malls and as a latchkey kid," Carolyn explained, as we began to talk. "My parents didn't return home until nine o'clock in the evenings. They both worked a lot. When I was nineteen, in 1995,

I moved to France. That was when I met a real family, the parents of my then boyfriend. Immediately I learned that every meal is a priority that deserves to be considered quality time. Sunday is a particularly important day that includes family, friends, and celebration. The meal is something to be treasured, taken in slowly, respected as the centerpiece of conversation and connectivity."

I wondered how difficult this adjustment might have been, given the independence of the typical young American woman, but Carolyn assured me that the transition was effortless as she quickly adapted to her new life. One of her fondest memories is of a baptism she attended that lasted more than fourteen hours. "The ritual at the church lasted about five or ten minutes," she remembered, laughing, "but the meal went on for the remainder of the day! There must have been twenty courses, and these were not wealthy people. We danced and lingered between dishes."

I sensed her delight in the memory and asked if she was bored or conscious of the time that passed. "Initially I thought, wow, we've been here for a while, but I loved it—the wine, the celebration. It was all very easy to embrace," she recalled. She looked forward to Sunday each week.

Before leaving for France, where she lived for four years, Carolyn had attended the University of Illinois, where a typical meal in the cafeteria was mac and cheese. When she enrolled in college in France, she instantly noticed that wine and beer were offered in the school cafeteria. "If wine and beer were available at the University of Illinois everyone would be wasted," she giggled. "But in France it was, like, it's there, no big deal. Moderation and appreciation are the mind-set, and that applies to food as much as to alcohol." Another revelation—fast food and refined food were nowhere to be found; in France, even truck stops offer fabulous food.

In Carolyn's new life in the Normandy region of France, fresh seafood and cream sauces, as well as food from her garden, took the place of take-out and frozen food. "The frozen-food aisle in the local grocery store offered few choices, whereas artisanal chesses and fresh fish were abundant," she recalled.

A typical day in France begins with breakfast, *le petit déjeuner*—often fresh, homemade jam on toast or a baguette with coffee. Children drink chocolate milk with their breakfast. Lunch, *le déjeuner*, is generally the main meal and can run to several courses; some shops close between 11:00 A.M. and 1:00 P.M. or 12 noon and 2:00 P.M., the shopkeepers returning home to prepare, cook, and enjoy lunch before going back to work. A sweet dessert is more commonly shared with guests than during daily family meals; however, several cheese offerings typically follow *le dîner* every evening.

Carolyn recounted her French boyfriend's reaction to Americans walking while eating. He'd never witnessed that in France and found it rather funny. In France, a meal was a special time that deserved one's full attention and respect.

I asked Carolyn if she had encountered anyone in France who dieted or mentioned dieting. Her answer: "Never."

"You might see a lighter supper on Sunday night after a large lunch, but that's as close as you'll come to a diet," she explained. And for exercise, she found that gardening, biking, walking, doing things outside, and just being outside are common activities, while exercise in a gym is not.

We discussed some of the differences between American and French women who become iconic figures. "There is no equivalent of Pamela Anderson in France. The French icon is very natural, refined, and neat—like Jane Birkin, an English actress and film director living in France. Jane is charismatic, inspiring, and influential and adored more than idealized or copied. The French don't worry about closing gapped teeth, and one-of-a-kind is the goal more than following the crowd," Carolyn stated.

I was very curious about whether Carolyn missed her home. "People in the United States are more casual, flexible, and up-front, and I like that. America is eclectic and multi-cultural, and I missed that diversity while living abroad."

Since her time in France, Carolyn has returned to the States and married an American. Today, with the help of her husband, she juggles her role as a mother of two small children and a demanding job as a hotel general manager.

"So how do you do it?" I asked. "Can you possibly recreate the life you enjoyed in France?"

Carolyn explained, "It has to be a *value*, and we do make the time to eat together as a family. I enjoy cooking, and although my meals are not as elaborate as I might have enjoyed in France, we do sit down together every evening to a meal prepared with quality ingredients. I maintain a vegetable garden—something I picked up in France.

"I still remember a quote that a friend shared with me in France. It's a statement by the eighteenth-century gastronome and writer Jean Anthelme Brillat-Savarin: 'He who receives his friends and gives no personal attention to the meal which is being prepared for them is not worthy of having friends.'

"I want to be a good friend," Carolyn adds, "so I'll continue to make my best effort to carry on all that I learned about food, friends, and family during my time in France!

Carolyn's time abroad taught her that the idea of quality is more far-reaching than just the good food the French eat. Quality of *life* is of great value in France; enjoying family and friends is cherished way above any quantity of possessions or any amount of wealth.

La Qualité au dessus de la Quantité:
Quality over Quantity

The world has changed from quality to quantity, and so have we.
—Santosh Kalwar

Dani stepped off the jetway at Chicago's O'Hare gripping an awkward, antiquated, olive-green suitcase in one hand. In the opposite arm she clutched a furry stuffed animal, along with other gifts from her native Bad Salzuflen, a town in the Lippe district of North Rhine–Westphalia, Germany.

Following a welcome celebration that centered around a homemade Black Forest cherry torte—a *Schwarzwälder Kirschtorte*, my entire German vocabulary—I helped Dani unpack. It dawned on me that this sixteen-year-old design student and fashionista carried a year's worth of clothing, shoes, and accessories in just one suitcase! As Dani thoughtfully unfolded her simple pink Benetton sweatshirt and placed it among her things, it was clear to me that every item she owned was chosen with the same care most teenage girls dedicate to the selection of a prom dress. Her suitcase held one of the best of everything.

In our world of superstores, supersized burgers and drinks, and warehouse clubs it's easy to get the whole concept turned around to something more like quantity, quantity, and more quantity over quality. When this mind-set persists, affecting the food we purchase, prepare, and consume, our suitcases *and* bellies overflow.

Whereas dieting lowers the boom, with this book I propose raising the bar.

The French eat a significantly greater amount of fat without the elevated levels of harmful cholesterol and heart disease that we Americans experience. This is because the *quality* of European food is substantially higher and the quantities (portions) consumed at a meal are substantially smaller.

I recall visiting Brussels and peering into the shiny glass case at the local *boucherie*. I didn't recognize the meat. After I asked what I was looking at, imagine my embarrassment when the butcher replied, "Pork chops." The bright, whitish organic meat looked nothing like the two-toned, pale pork that I'm accustomed to here in the United States.

Elevate the quality of your food, and you will naturally eat less because high-quality, nutrient-dense food delivers the vitamins, minerals, and nutrients we need to feel satisfied. Eating poor-quality, nutrient-deficient food is like trying to fill a bottomless black hole—it just can't be done. Your body and brain working together sense the deficiencies, and before you know it a survival strategy kicks in, leaving you hungry for more.

In many other countries, including France, high-quality, whole food is the first line of defense in preventative health care. The purest vitamins and minerals are to be found at the local market; the finest medication is served on your plate.

The French reject supplements and the vitamin craze (except for that cellulite tonic you see in *la pharmacie*), reasoning that if you eat fresh foods why would you need vitamins? Eat a real yellow bell pepper and get your vitamin C; put spinach in your quiche, for God's sake, and get iron. Very sensible, indeed, if you live in France. The food there is so fresh you have to shake off the insects and dirt. Outside of Paris chances are good that your beef was mooing hours before being served up on the plate.

Europeans fanatically legislate the labeling of genetically modified foods. In Europe, food comes from the soil, not from a factory.

But in the States it's quite a different story, and even though we nutritionists recommend that people get their vitamins and minerals from food, I fear most of us do in fact need to fill the gaps in our diet through vitamin and mineral supplements. In addition to hit-or-miss eating and a diet lacking in vegetables, fruits, and whole grains, modern processing techniques have considerably reduced the vitamin and mineral content of many foods.

Add eating junk food to the mix and we become deficient in vitamins and subject to a host of attendant health problems. Medications taken to treat illnesses and conditions may deplete or inhibit the absorption of certain nutrients as well. For example, the use of oral contraceptives leaves women susceptible to low levels of vitamin C, folic acid, magnesium, zinc, and vitamins B2, B6, and B12.

Keeping It Fresh, and What to Do If You Can't

The length of time that fruits and veggies stay on the vine, ground, or tree has a major effect on two key aspects of their quality: their nutrient content and their flavor. The longer foods are able to ripen naturally, the higher the level of the nutrients they deliver and, usually, the richer their taste.

Unless you are choosing fresh produce from a farmers' market or your own backyard, chances are good that your produce was picked at least several days in advance and is not at its peak ripeness (otherwise it would spoil too quickly en route to the store). Also some of its nutritional value has undoubtedly degraded since it was picked, including during transport. Once fresh fruits and vegetables are harvested, they undergo higher rates of respiration—a physiologic process in which plant starches and sugars are converted into carbon dioxide, water, and other by-products; respiration leads to moisture loss, reduced quality, and susceptibility to bacterial spoilage.

Refrigeration during transport helps to slow the deterioration, but still, by the time you eat a fresh vegetable that has traveled across continents to reach your dinner table, a substantial amount of its nutritional value may be lost. This is why the "eat local" (aka locavore) movement is growing so rapidly.

It's a double-edged sword. Global shipping offers us access to fruits and vegetables we might not be able to get in the States, as well as sometimes lower prices. It also allows us to enjoy most fruits and veggies year-round, instead of just seasonally. But nutrient loss and diminished flavor are the obvious trade-offs.

Cool It

Produce destined for freezing is picked at its maximal ripeness, quickly frozen to a temperature at which it retains the most nutritional value and flavor, and kept frozen as it travels to the freezer in your local store. While there is some initial nutrient loss with the first steps in the freezing process—washing, peeling, and heat-based blanching (done for vegetables, but usually not fruits)—freezing keeps produce good for up to a year on average.

When you thaw, prepare, and eat frozen vegetables and fruits, you are getting most of the food's original nutritional value. Be assured, for example, that if you love blueberries and all of their health benefits, the frozen version is just as good as the fresh. (I happen to think that frozen fruits whip up into much better smoothies than fresh fruits.) And depending on how you cook or prepare the food, the dish may taste quite similar to one made with its fresh counterpart, or maybe even better.

Can It

The process is somewhat different for canned produce, where in some cases a food's nutritional value may suffer. As with freezing, the produce to be canned is picked at its maximal ripeness, blanched (though longer than for freezing), and then canned. In the case of spinach, sweet red peppers, cabbage, broccoli, asparagus, and other produce that contains water-soluble nutrients (which are most sensitive to heat loss) such as vitamin C and vitamin B1, an increased nutrient loss of 50 to 80 percent occurs during canning; losses of most other vitamins range from 10 to 30 percent.

Often fruit is canned in sugary syrup or juice, and salt is added to many vegetables to help enhance their flavor and avoid spoilage. These additions can make a very healthy fruit or vegetable much less desirable when canned than its fresh or frozen counterpart. But if the canning process is done without the addition of salt, sugar, or other ingredients (sauces, for example, for vegetables), in general the nutritional value of canned fruits and vegetables is similar to that of freshly and locally picked and frozen produce.

Look for canned fruit that is "in its own juice." For vegetables, check the sodium content on the nutritional label and aim for vegetables with "no added salt" and without butter or cream sauces. Because the canned produce is maintained in an oxygen-free environment, canned foods can last for years—but be wary of cans that are dented (a dent can include a tiny hole that can admit bacteria) or bulging (something bad is going on within).

According to the Food Network's Alton Brown, one of the smartest film directors I represented in my career as a film agent: "Because the sugar in peas quickly converts into starch, peas are picked and preserved at the height of their quality. In fact, peas were one of the first successes that Clarence Birdseye had in his experiments involving flash-freezing vegetables." Tune in to Alton's show, *Good Eats*, for education and entertainment on the science of food along with a dose of pop culture and a lot of wit and wisdom.

Is Fresh Always Best?

A single-minded approach to freshness, in my opinion, will do more harm than good. But what is better than fresh? Sometimes frozen, and sometimes even canned.

If you live in, say, California, near the farmers and the food, fresh is great and readily available.

But if you live in South Dakota, in the winter you'll be eating a lot of potatoes and parsnips and not much else. In this case, frozen and canned produce is a fresher, more sensible alternative. And even when a local farmer happens to offer fresh produce in your region, a can of stewed tomatoes or beans in the pantry are a cook's dream and sometimes even a healthier nutritional choice when the urge for homemade vegetable soup strikes.

Here are some examples of how specific nutrients are affected by canning and freezing. Yes, it takes a bit of effort to take in all of this detailed information, but the payoff will be produce on your plate that tastes terrific and delivers all the benefits it's capable of.*

Vitamin C. Vitamin C is sensitive to heat, light, and oxygen. Fresh produce stored at the appropriate temperature and consumed within a relatively short period of time is the best source of vitamin C. But in produce stored for too long, vitamin C degrades rapidly. Vitamin C is also lost with blanching—though some fruits with ascorbic acid (like oranges, lemons, grapefruits, and limes) that undergo freezing may retain more vitamin C than even the fresh stuff. And unfortunately, a large percentage of vitamin C is lost with the initial canning process.

Here's a kitchen preparation tip offering convenience as well as a maximum dose of vitamin C. Squeeze a dozen fresh lemons, discarding the seeds, and pour the juice into ice cube trays, filling them almost to the top. Freeze until firm (the lemon juice will never totally solidify). Pop out the individual "cubes" as you need them for recipes. I like to add a cube of lemon juice to some of my salad dressings, sauces for meats and veggies, and even my lentil soup.

B Vitamins. Most B vitamins are sensitive to heat and light, which means that there is significant loss of these vitamins when produce is blanched before being frozen or canned. Again, fresh produce tends to be the best source for this vitamin group.

Polyphenolic Compounds. Water-soluble polyphenolic compounds, which are rich in beneficial antioxidants—they inhibit oxidation in the body and thus prevent damage to healthy cells—can be found in the skins of peaches, pears, and apples, but are lower in products that are frozen or canned without the skin. When the skin or the natural juice is included in the can, levels of polyphenols are as high or higher in canned produce compared with fresh.

Fat-soluble Vitamin A and Carotenoids and Vitamin E. Little fat-soluble vitamin content is lost in blanching, so in general frozen and canned are just as good as fresh for these nutrients. However, there can be some losses or even gains, depending on the specific fruit or vegetable. For example, fresh green beans have more beta-carotene than frozen or canned green beans, but frozen peas have more beta-carotene than either fresh or canned, and canned tomatoes have the highest levels of beta-carotene and lycopene, most likely due to release of those nutrients with the heat of the blanching process.

Minerals, Fiber, Carbohydrates, Proteins, and Fats. Levels of these nutrients are similar in fresh, canned, and frozen fruits and vegetables.

To learn more about the benefits of all fruits and vegetables, whether fresh, frozen, or canned, as well as for food tips, recipes, and interactive tools, go to www.fruitsandveggiesmatter.gov.

Shopping like the French

It is common for the French to buy cheese from the *fromagerie*, bread from the *boulangerie*, meat from the *boucherie*, and fruits and vegetables from the open-air *marché*. It is more time-consuming and sometimes more expensive than picking everything up at one time from the supermarket, but the products are fresher and of better quality.

It wasn't until we moved to New York City and had access to exceptional boutique food stores that I fully understood the value of selecting each food in this manner. Now I find it impossible to buy a slice of cheese at the supermarket when I know that my cheese man, Kevin, is right around the corner with a wheel of brie ripening on the counter. Just the other night I ran in to see Kevin for a block of cheese that was essential to a recipe I was preparing.

"Are you using it tonight?" he asked.

"Yes, in just a little while," I answered, curious.

"Good. Cheese must not be cold. You can't taste it that way. Leave it out of the refrigerator," he ordered.

Carol's French Kitchen
MON GARDE-MANGER (MY PANTRY)

High-quality, cold-pressed extra-virgin olive oil
Reims champagne vinegar
Jean LeBlanc aged balsamic vinegar
Maille Dijon mustard
Fleur de sel (sea salt) for finishing vegetables and meats
French green and black peppercorns
Herbes de Provence
Fresh pistachios
Local honey
Provence black fig jam
Chantaine orange marmalade
St. Dalfour wild blueberry jam
Rosemary and olive oil crackers
Individually wrapped sugar cubes from France (bought online
from www.poshchicago.com)
Valrhona French chocolate squares (bought in bulk online at
www.worldwidechocolate.com)

CHAMPAGNE VINAIGRETTE

2 teaspoons Dijon mustard
1/4 cup champagne vinegar
3/4 cup extra-virgin olive oil
1/2 teaspoon salt
Pinch of freshly ground black pepper

In a small bowl, combine mustard and vinegar; whisk together. While whisking constantly, slowly drizzle in olive oil. Season with salt and pepper. The vinaigrette may be stored in the refrigerator in an airtight container for up to 1 month. Makes 1 cup.

To make homemade champagne vinegar, simply store leftover champagne in an open, wide-mouthed jar at room temperature. Within a few weeks, the wine will have turned to vinegar.

MON FRIGO (MY FRIDGE)

San Pellegrino Sparkling Natural Mineral Water

A bottle of French champagne

A smooth, velvety goat's milk French Brie

Parmigiano Reggiano

Fresh black and green olive mix

Organic walnuts and almonds (stored in the *frigo* for freshness)

Organic arugula

Fresh organic basil, thyme, and parsley

Greek yogurt

Vegetarian-fed omega-3 enriched eggs

Organic milk

Organic, salted, fresh cream butter

Organic apples (we like them sliced and chilled with Brie or Parmigiano Reggiano)

SUR LE COMPTOIR (ON MY COUNTERTOP)

Organic avocado

Organic garlic cloves

Shallots

Organic heirloom tomatoes

When we dined that evening I slowed down to take special note and greater pleasure in the nutty essence of the creamy cheese Kevin had so respectfully procured. I'm not sure that would have been the case had it not been for a quick chat with my cheese man.

Lucky for me, now that I live in New York I am able to shop at the French bakery for bread and the butcher for meat. But if you live in an area where you don't have access to specialty shopping or a farmers' market, don't be discouraged. Epicurean food items abound on the Internet. And stop in to meet the baker and the butcher in your local supermarket. I haven't met a baker who doesn't take pride in his bread or a butcher who isn't happy to share her expertise on the subject of the right meat cuts for preparing the perfect French beef bourguignon.

Mind and Meals Over Makeup

The old saying "You are what you eat" is a long-established scientific fact. So while the French woman supplements her diet with a few facials each month, she faithfully holds to the belief that the very best way to augment her looks is with the beauty foods of nature. For luminous skin, strong nails, shiny hair, and brilliant eyes the French woman works from the inside out, enjoying a wide variety of only the highest-quality seasonal fresh fruits and vegetables.

The desire for radiant skin may be the only true fixation of the typical French woman. While Americans, including myself, tend to approach personal skin care with efficiency, French women regard the treatment of the skin, hair, and body as an enjoyable, rewarding ritual.

Outside of the facial fixation, French women pride themselves on being more balanced than Americans. They see America as a youth-obsessed, throwaway, quick-fix culture where women look artificial and "done."

French women steer clear of excessive makeup. The French attitude is that makeup will only accumulate in the creases that come with age and make one look older. And using too much makeup means you are hiding from yourself.

Consider French politician Ségolène Royal. She wears almost no makeup, but when she had an upper tooth straightened in 2005, the daily newspaper *Libération* was horrified. "The French people's favorite Socialist is now endowed with an American smile," *Libération* wrote.

In the United States, we marvel at Catherine Deneuve, whereas in France she is an object of pity as a result of her obvious facial interventions and made-up face. "Poor Catherine," said Terry de Gunzenurg, creator of the *By Terry* makeup line. "She let herself get hooked by the syndrome of Dorian Gray, of eternal youth. It's sad."*

Staying Beautiful from the Inside Out: Body and Beauty Foods

Let food be your medicine and medicine be your food.

—Hippocrates

French or American, we are all well served by a nutrient-dense diet. And there are a few foods that pack more than their share of nutrients and phytochemicals that protect our health from the inside out, lowering women's risks for diseases such as breast cancer and heart disease and keeping us beautiful along the way!

For a comprehensive listing of what we in the nutrition community consider the essential body and beauty foods, see this book's Appendix. Meanwhile, as a sampler, sink your teeth into the top ten face-friendly foods.

Dark Leafy Greens: Acne Attackers

Brilliantly deep leafy greens like spinach and kale are full of antioxidants, and they're a great source of iron. Dark circles under your eyes? You're probably not getting enough iron. The same goes for acne. A 1977 Swedish study on the effects of zinc on acne consisted of 64 acne patients who were divided into four groups and given either a zinc supplement or a placebo. After only four weeks on zinc therapy, 65 percent of those given a zinc supplement were clearly improved; after 12 weeks, 87 percent were totally in the clear. The evidence was overwhelming. To quote the Swedish study, zinc's effect on acne is "remarkable." Those in the study took 45 mg of zinc, three times per day.*

Olive Oil: Dryness Defeater

Aiming for smooth, supple skin? Dermatologists recommend that women with persistently dry, flaky skin eat more high-quality fats—those found in olive oil and other monounsaturated oils like sesame oil—as well as foods containing healthy fats, such as avocados and walnuts. Adding just a tablespoon of healthy oils to the daily diet will result in noticeable improvement in as little as a few weeks. Even women with clogged pores who regularly eat these foods will benefit from their essential fatty acids, which help keep the pores clear by thinning the oils they secrete.

Water: Moisture Booster

How do you know if you're dehydrated? Just look in the mirror. Is your skin ashen and gray? That's what dehydration looks like. Instead of rushing off to the dermatologist's office for a round of dermal fillers to plump up your drooping jowls, try hydrating first. Water is the first line of defense for dull, droopy skin because it makes existing winkles look less obvious. To see results, though, you need a substantial amount of H_2O every day. Make sure to down about half of your body weight in ounces daily (a 120-pound woman will drink 60 ounces)—even more if you work out.

Ripe Tomatoes: Skin Elasticizers

A simple slice or two of tomato on your sandwich packs high levels of the antioxidant vitamins A and C, as well as chemicals that fight skin cancer. Vitamin A aids in healing acne from the inside out by boosting your immune system and helping to resist infection. Vitamin C keeps skin elastic and prevents bruising. You'll also get these antioxidants in other dark red, orange, and yellow fruits and vegetables.

Berries: Wrinkle Fighters

You've heard all the talk about berries, and it's true: Berries are a great source of polyphenols, antioxidants touted for their anti-aging capabilities. Blueberries, raspberries, strawberries, and blackberries are among the fruits that have been shown to protect short-term memory and balance. A mere half cup of blueberries is packed with three times the antioxidants a large orange delivers. A handful of strawberries yields all the antioxidant vitamin C your body requires each day to reconstruct your collagen, the framework that keeps the jowls from drooping.

Salmon: Inflammation Calmer

Salmon, one of the fattiest of all fish (and I mean this in the best possible way), is packed with face-friendly omega-3 fatty acids, which do everything from moisturize parched areas of your skin to help shrink red-looking pimples. And don't forget about mackerel, bass, and trout, as the essential fatty acids in these foods also combat collagen-damaging free radicals and help smooth out fine lines. I eat salmon three times a week. If you don't like seafood, a fish-oil supplement offers some of the same benefits. Or try adding flaxseed oil and nuts to your diet. Fatty fish and nuts also contain zinc, which helps suppress acne break-outs and increase cell rejuvenation.

Cantaloupes: Flakiness Foilers

Sweet-tasting, sunny-colored cantaloupe is full of compounds like lycopene, which reduces the collagen damage that promotes wrinkles. Skin sage Dr. N. V. Perricone often prescribes cantaloupe to drab-skinned patients. Cantaloupe, especially the light flesh just underneath the skin, is a great source of beta-carotene, so be sure to scoop that up. This fleshy fruit is just what the skin needs to prevent dry rough patches on the backs of the arms as well as acne cysts.

Soybeans: Pimple Opponents

If you're struggling with acne, dermatologists recommend sending the soybean to the rescue. Soybeans are full of nutrients that act like estrogen, and they are loaded with vitamin E, which enhances new cell growth and keeps skin hydrated. My prescription? Go for at least half a cup of soy in the form of beans two to three times a week. It's important to note that tofu and soymilk, even though they are soybean products, are processed foods. Whenever possible, make the healthier choice of eating the whole food. Keep processed food to a minimum for optimum health—and pimple protection.

Carrots: Wrinkle Wranglers

What's up, Doc? That wascally wabbit was right—carrots are full of the beta-carotene your body turns into vitamin A, the vitamin that says bye-bye to dry, flaky skin. And it's not only carrots that deliver this benefit; several other orange fruits and vegetables—apricots, papaya, pumpkin, mango, and sweet potatoes—are also great skin savers.

Oatmeal: Toxin Ouster

Fiber is your friend! When it comes to the fiber in oatmeal, go for the slow-cooked kind, not the instant. You'll get a hefty dose of fiber that, once converted, helps filter toxins and guarantee a clearer complexion. Oatmeal is also rich in the B vitamins, which aid new skin-cell growth.

A Tale of the Table: *Babette's Feast*

The story in the film *Babette's Feast* takes place in the fall of 1871. After fleeing a French civil war in which her husband and son were executed, Babette had arrived with nothing but a letter of introduction in a small village in Denmark, where she became the maid and cook for Martine and Philippa, sisters who preside over a small, strict Lutheran sect founded by their father. They have lived lives of piety and work among the poor.

In France Babette had operated a fine restaurant, but as the film opens she has spent the last fourteen years as a domestic servant, preparing staple meals of split cod and ale-bread.

Martine and Philippa are planning a simple celebration for what would have been their father's 100th birthday, when Babette is notified that she has won ten thousand francs in the French lottery. She decides that in gratitude to the sisters and the village, she will spend the money on preparing a fancy French meal for them.

After reluctantly giving their permission, the sisters are amazed at the foods she buys, including turtle, live quail, and expensive wines. The feast consists of the finest dishes and wines served at Café Anglais, Babette's restaurant in Paris.

Potage a'la tortue (turtle soup)
Blini Demidoff au Caviar (buckwheat cakes with caviar)
Caille en sarcophage avec sauce perigourdine (quail in
puff-pastry shell with foie gras and truffle sauce)
La salade (salad)
Les fromages (cheese and fresh fruit)
Baba au rhum avec les figues (rum cake with dried figs)

After a prayer, the dinner begins. The wine is opened and poured, the turtle soup ladled into each bowl. Next, tiny pancakes garnished with odd-looking, fishy-smelling little black eggs—caviar! And champagne! And then as the guests begin to sip another glass of vintage wine, the aroma of something special wafts through the dining room: *caille en sarcophage avec sauce perigourdine*. It is a masterpiece—tender, gamey quail stuffed with *foie gras* and encased in a puff-pastry shell, swimming in a pool of black truffles hand-picked in the Perigord region of France. Rare bottles of Clos de Vougeot are poured into crystal goblets. Dinner ends with a fabulous rum cake with *glaceé* and fresh fruits.

Most summaries of *Babette's Feast* explore its many themes, ranging from politics to religion to art. But I am preoccupied with the food, which for me is as central to this great film as any of its characters, events, or ideas. One of the guests, General Loewenhielm, speaks of the first time he had experienced the feast's main dish:

> One day in Paris, after I had won a riding competition, my French fellow officers invited me out to dine at one of the finest restaurants, the Café Anglais. The chef, surprisingly enough, was a woman. We were served *caille en sarcophage*, a dish of her own creation. General Galliffet, who was our host for the evening, explained that this woman, the head chef, had the ability to transform a dinner into a kind of love affair, a love affair that made no distinction between bodily appetite and spiritual appetite. General Galliffet said that in the past he had fought a duel for the love of a beautiful woman. But now there was no woman in Paris for whom he would shed his blood—except this chef. She was considered the greatest culinary genius. What we are now eating is nothing less than *caille en sarcophage*.

The writer and director focus on the culinary sequence from beginning to end, on Babette's insistence on and procurement of the finest French ingredients, on the labor-intensive transporting of the ingredients to the kitchen and ultimately the table, on the details of the cooking and serving, and finally on the magical effect of a feast that can make the most rigid and solemn diners ready to shed their blood for the chef. This feast is truly a love affair that makes no distinction between bodily and spiritual appetite.

PRACTICING YOUR FRENCH

This week:

1. Upgrade three foods that you eat on a regular basis. For example, if you routinely eat iceberg lettuce, upgrade to romaine. If you eat romaine lettuce, upgrade to arugula.
2. Choose from only the outside perimeter of the supermarket. For the next week, eliminate all foods packaged in a box or a bag, opting only for whole foods. Enjoy an apple in place of apple sauce, edamame (fresh soy beans) in place of soy milk, fresh peanuts instead of peanut butter. For the next week get back in touch with unadulterated food.

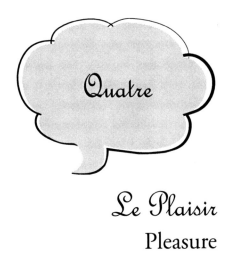

Quatre

Le Plaisir
Pleasure

Life itself is the proper binge.
—*Julia Child*

I'M NORMALLY NOT an envious person, but I'll admit right here and now that in 1998 when Susan told me that she and her husband were spending the next two years in Paris I turned a little green.

A few years earlier, when I was in the film business, my pal Mark Falls and I had worked with Susan, a freelance broadcast television producer. Mark was the creative director for the same post-production facility in Atlanta where I was director of sales. In 1998 Mark and I had ended up in Belgium for business, and I was hoping we would find our way to Paris and check in with Susan.

Our objective was to secure a contract to design, create, and execute a new station identity for the CNN equivalent RTL TVI in Brussels. Our contact there, François, a French-speaking Belgian from the southern region of Wallonia, admired the appearance of American television, particularly the colorful station-identification logos and banners. It was quite an honor even to be considered for this project, and over the course of several meetings and meals and though suffering from jet lag, we won the contract, along with a wonderful long-term relationship with François.

As many things as we Americans love about the French, the French appreciate many of our qualities as well. François was quite taken with Mark's out-of-the-box ingenuity, as well as the intense tenacity, dedication, and drive of Americans. And of course, our great television logos and banners!

Once our business was finished in Belgium, we tossed a coin—heads it's Paris, tails Amsterdam. Heads it was, so we ended up in Paris and called Susan. Unfortunately, she was already committed to other activities, but she did manage to impress us with her telephone French before we hit the streets without her.

Ooh la la! I had been hoping for Paris! No longer on an expense account, we had opted to take the train to get there, and once we arrived, Mark insisted we take public transportation everywhere—just for fun. Didn't sound like fun to me, but I've always been a pushover for Mark, a big teddy bear of a guy, so I went along. Besides, he knew a little bit more French than I did, a very little bit.

We arrived at the Saint-Lazare station to a reception line of French soldiers bearing some serious ammunition. A little unsettled at best, we swept by them; they were like statues, one after the other in their camouflage, and they never flinched. I wondered if Amsterdam would have seemed more welcoming.

After sucking in a deep breath of train station fumes, I trailed Mark until I figured out that I had tracked him in a complete circle. There we were, face to face with the soldiers, again. Now I think they *were* flinching. Mark gave me a wide-open eyeball that I knew meant keep going and act cool. Then we completed the loop *again.* The soldiers were looking at us now, *suspiciously!*

The heck with Mark's ego, I decided. "Where is the exit?" I pleaded to the glaring statues. I wasn't sure they were allowed to respond, so I was a bit startled when one rifle-toting Frenchman pointed the way. He certainly wasn't Officer Friendly, but I'm sure he was at least partially amused at our lame directional skills. We couldn't even find our way out of the station.

We climbed the concrete stairway. Sunlight glistened in waves as we walked a few short blocks until suddenly we stood before the Opéra Garnier. A lump formed in my throat as tears filled my eyes, which were now fixed on this building crowning the Avenue de l'Opéra. I relished an uninterrupted vision of the monument; I suspected that the street had been cleared of trees in order to offer passersby unusual access to the unobstructed and glorious scene.

A long whiff of griddled crepe batter, laced with vanilla, from the take-away stand on the opposite corner enlivened all of my senses. Around the corner from the Opéra Garnier was the Café de le Paix, where people sat side by side, spectator style, so that each person could enjoy the excellent people-watching. Like magic—as though from night to day, without dusk in between—we had been transported to one of the liveliest districts in the heart of Paris, where street after street was devoted to shopping.

After several minutes of silence, during which I avoided Mark's gaze for fear of emotional overload, I glanced his way. He looked as awestruck as I was, which helped me feel less conspicuous. I vowed mutely to return with the love of my life, and I suspect that Mark was having the identical thought.

Without a word we walked and gawked and walked. Mark to this day calls it the death march because we walked through arrondissement after arrondissement for more than twelve hours. We did stop for lunch, where Mark started to complain about his aching feet—until he tasted his first bite of fruit salad. The fruit was so fresh and exploding with flavor that he looked at me inquisitively, as if tasting fruit for the first time: "What is this food? I've never known it before." Reaching across the table, stabbing the fruit with my fork, I understood his reaction. "How can it be," I marveled, "that fruit can taste so distinctive?"

Savourez le Goût: Savor the Flavor

It was during this first trip to Europe that I experienced the art of dining rather than eating and discovered the fourth secret of the French woman: the benefits of indulging in the pleasures that food offers.

Mark and I had always enjoyed lunching together; he had a palate that appreciated fine cuisine, while I conformed as best I could to the limitations of my current diet. This trip expanded both of our culinary horizons with some extraordinary meals— for example, the lunch our client, François, had arranged for us in Brussels on our first day working together.

Under a radiant summer sun, we dined outdoors under umbrellas that I would have pictured in Nice or Cannes. The café was quaint, with a provincial feel, and I was amazed that such a feast could be prepared in its modest kitchen. We lingered over lunch, which seemed peculiar to me given the deadlines Mark and I were anticipating for accomplishing the project we had just signed up for. But to judge from François's demeanor as he licked the pâté from his chops and ordered the next of many courses, we had all the time in the world.

One of my first courses was a simple endive salad, nothing fancy yet so wonderful that I had to ask our waiter what made it so scrumptious. "It's the dressing," he explained in almost perfect English. "The champagne vinegar is the secret, then extra-virgin olive oil, but especially lots of sea salt." Mark shared a bit of his salmon tartar while we anticipated our main dish, *sole meunière.*

AN AMERICAN IN PARIS: EATING 101—SIT AND ENJOY

At the start of this chapter, I talk about my American friend Susan, who lived in Paris for two years. She couldn't meet up with me and my pal Mark when we made an unplanned trip—my first—to the city. You can imagine my delight, as I did research for this book twelve years later, when Susan agreed to give me some perspective on her French experience. In this special section and others in the following chapters, all titled "An American in Paris," Susan talks about various aspects of her life in the City of Light.

"How about rituals, the rhythms of life—what stands out?" I began.

"The French visit the market twice a day for fresh bread. An older woman who lived in my building walked to the patisserie for her fresh demi-baguette every morning and afternoon. If I were out walking Gracie, my Labrador, she would offer her a little taste," Susan recalled.

"Also, the French sit and eat. One rarely sees a French person with a sandwich in their hand dashing off to catch a cab. You'll never catch them eating in their cars like Americans often do. Even though *food rapid* is available and there is a McDonalds on the Champs Elysées, the French sit and eat. There are far more tables in the McDonalds in Paris then I have ever seen in the States. The French enjoy their food, while Americans see it as an afterthought, if a thought at all," she said.

"Americans eat and run," Susan explained. "When eating out in the States, the meal is over in forty-five minutes, if that. Heavy appetizers served before the entrée crush the palate before the main meal arrives. In Paris, when you dine out, relaxing for hours at the table is expected; the waiter never rushes you to 'turn over' the table to others who are waiting to be seated. Meals in Paris are for relaxing and enjoying, and sitting in an outdoor café or by a window and watching people walk by is like having your own little theater right in front of you. Meals in America seem to be for the sole purpose of efficiency, not to enjoy the food."

The fish came to the table whole, with the head on, in a sheer sauce of browned butter and lemon juice, topped with chopped parsley and with a half-dozen peeled potatoes standing by. The lemon kicked its way through the richness of that nutty butter sauce, which I adored. I fell hard for that *sole meunière*!

This luxurious meal (lunch is the most important meal of the day in Belgium) lasted more than two hours—long enough for us to savor, digest, and assimilate food prepared with the finest ingredients, including pride and lots of passion. The Belgians are fond of saying that their food is cooked with French finesse and served in portions of German generosity. It's no wonder that it took almost no effort for me to adapt to this new pace. My love affair with *sole meunière* and all French food that's taken in pleasure, relaxation, and reverence continues to this day.

Imagine my delight years later when finally I connected the dots and discovered that pleasure in dining is a wonderful weight-management secret!

The French do not rush to the rescue when their stomachs first rumble. They actually feel the hunger pangs and sense the body's cues. There's a saying that goes back to the ancient Romans: "Hunger is the best sauce." As the French see it today, the longer the wait, the sweeter the return. They sit down, stay seated, enjoy, and *savor* every bite, unlike Americans, who tend to view mealtime as fast and functional.

Our French friends love their food, but not the way Americans love food. The French are more gourmets, while we Americans are, truth to tell, pretty much gluttons. We confuse enjoyment of food with over-consumption.

Rather than pile several foods on the plate or the fork at once, the French enjoy courses one after the other, independently. The result: Only 39 percent of Americans claim to greatly enjoy eating, compared to 90 percent of people in France.

In this country, it's not unusual to see someone shoving down a hamburger and fries while working on a laptop, driving a car, talking on a cell phone, watching TV, even walking down the street. Americans have a relationship with food that often excludes joy and pleasure—and makes us eat more.

Unlike the majority of Americans, the French eat until their hunger is satisfied, not until they are "stuffed." Enjoying a meal in a leisurely fashion helps you know when to stop eating because you've had enough. It takes around 15 minutes for your brain to get the message that your stomach is full, so eating slowly makes it more likely you'll stop when you're satisfied as opposed to way too full. Conversely, eating quickly makes it easy to overshoot the mark and walk away from the table with an uncomfortably stretched stomach.

In an international study* groups of people from different countries were asked questions dealing with their beliefs about the link between diet and health and their concerns about food. The group that associated food most with health and least with pleasure was the Americans, and the most pleasure-oriented and least health-oriented group was the French.

It's one thing to draw an intuitive conclusion that the French are slimmer because they savor and enjoy their food during two-hour lunches that involve interesting conversation and the sipping of wine, but it's another thing altogether when scientific studies back up that notion. When I read the research on the study I am about to share with you in Marc David's book *The Slow Down Diet*, the whole nutritional universe as I knew it changed. In fact, his influence as a nutritionist specializing in the psychology of eating motivated me to learn more about the practices of the French and ultimately share this knowledge with you.

Researchers from Sweden and Thailand determined how cultural preferences for food (in other words, the enjoyment people feel from eating the food) affect the absorption of iron from a meal.* A group of women from each country was fed the typical Thai meal—rice, veggies, coconut, fish sauce, and hot chili paste. Thai women enjoy Thai food, but many Swedish women don't.

This proved to be a critical metabolic fact, because even though the meals all contained the same amount of iron, the Swedish women absorbed only half as much iron as the Thai women. To complete this stage of the study, both groups received a typical Swedish meal—hamburger, mashed potatoes, and string beans, and again each meal contained the same amount of iron. The Thai women absorbed notably less iron from the Swedish meal.

Taste and pleasure are more essential to life than we could have ever imagined. Here's my take-away . . . When I savor a chocolate meringue, I will be completely guilt free!

Amanda's Story

"I say *France*, you say . . ."

"Taking it easy," my friend Amanda giggled. "Before arriving in Paris I was on medication for a digestive issue. Within a day or so of being in France, I looked at my husband, Jed, and said, I don't think I have to take these pills anymore. Like that, my stomach issues resolved." As I listened to the story of Amanda's trip to France, I was impressed by how quickly slowing down, relaxing, calmly digesting, and enjoying meals improved Amanda's well-being.

"For two weeks, while in Paris and then Le Thor, a small town on the banks of the Sorgue, I discontinued my prescription pills and felt physically better than I had in months," Amanda reminisced. "The stomach pain and the burning were gone."

Amanda shared an illuminating story about her first dining-out experience in Paris. "My friend took us to a special restaurant. She dropped us off, but before she left, she ordered for us. I remember the meal, a beautiful pork chop with a gorgeous purple potato on top—so simple, yet stunning. I propped my bum on the edge of the chair and inhaled it. Jed did, too. We often laugh about this; when we're into our food we don't speak to each other while we're eating.

"Midway through the meal I commented to Jed that the waiter never checked back with us. Despite this observation, we continued gulping our food. A few moments passed, and here we were—ready to go! Experience the city—let's get on with it! The waiter stood a mere ten feet away and still didn't make eye contact. Finally, I sat back, looked at Jed, and said, 'Why are we in such a hurry?'

"All I can say is, thank God this happened the first night. I looked at my fellow diners, relaxed, dining, savoring. It struck me that this is such a different way of life, far more than just a personal choice. All of the elements that surround the French contribute to this lifestyle. In a U.S. restaurant, I'm constantly aware that people are waiting for our table; the server rushes you away with the check. The whole setting is manic, making it almost impossible to savor the experience.

"Our eyes were suddenly open to our bad habits in the U.S. I remember the pancakes I made for a friend who dropped by during the breakfast hour. He was on the run, so he grabbed the pancake, folded it in half, and ate it in two bites. He was eating unconsciously, and so was I," Amanda admitted.

"Still, when I saw feathers on the farm-fresh eggs we were about to eat in France I was taken aback. But then I thought, at least I know where this egg is coming from. In our stores at home the Styrofoam package tells you about the eggs, but who knows how to interpret what's printed there?

"In Le Thor we stayed with friends who treated us like royalty. Despite our pleas to be allowed to treat them to a meal out, they shopped and prepared a meal that was unfamiliar to us: duck, sliced peaches, and peach cream sauce. I thought, if I have to eat this, I'll shoot myself. Next thing you know I'm scraping the plate with my fork, lapping up every drop. It was simply delicious. And fresh baguettes at every meal—I only wish I could find a baguette of that quality here in the States."

"Amanda, in your opinion as a wife and working mother, can you possibly reconstruct and sustain the French lifestyle, if not a simple baguette?" I inquired.

"You lose it quickly," she answered, "because you get caught up in the chaos of our everyday lives here. I have tried to re-create some of the meals we enjoyed there, but that's impossible due to the differences in food quality."

Once home, Amanda and Jed took off for the open-air farmers' market in their neighborhood. Upon inquiring, however, they learned that not one item at the

RUNAWAY BRIDE

In the movie *Runaway Bride* Maggie Carpenter (played by Julia Roberts) becomes so involved in her fiancé of the moment that her identity changes like the colors of a chameleon. As she loses touch with herself, she becomes increasingly afraid of marriage, gets cold feet, and runs. Maggie has left three men at the altar. As she prepares for a wedding with her fourth groom-to-be, we meet writer Ike Graham (Richard Gere), who is working on a story about her failed attempts to tie the knot. When Ike and Maggie become romantically involved, he makes her face her fears and herself.

> IKE
>
> That's right. You're so lost you don't even know how you like your eggs.
>
> MAGGIE
>
> What!?
>
> IKE
>
> With the priest, you liked them scrambled. With the Dead Head, fried. With the bug guy, poached. Now it's egg whites only, thank you very much.
>
> MAGGIE
>
> That's called changing your mind.
>
> IKE
>
> No, that's called not having a mind of your own.

Later in the film Maggie goes through an elaborate taste test with a spread of eggs prepared every way imaginable. She reports back to Ike.

> MAGGIE
>
> Eggs Benedict—I *love* eggs Benedict.

Whether you want a way of eating or a life partner, you must know your own mind. Be happy, accepting, honest, and realistic—about yourself, first and foremost. Scrutinize your life and your identity in order to know what you like, and what you can and cannot live with or without.

market was grown nearby. There were a few local companies offering fruit, but when they asked where the fruit came from, the merchant replied, "I haven't got a clue." Upon further inspection Amanda discovered that the fruit was not even from this country. In all, 95 percent of the products offered at the market were *not local*. (Not all farmers' market are created equal. Check out www.localharvest.org for locally grown produce in your area.)

As you might have guessed, Amanda is once again taking prescription pills for her digestive problems. One thing has changed, though; when she visits her local bakery, she has a completely different feeling about the man who bakes the bread. "In France I learned that it is an honor to make bread, a substance so basic to sustaining life. Previously, I had disregarded the importance of this contribution, but now I have deep respect for the profession."

Turned On by Food

In his book *The Slow Down Diet*, nutritionist Marc David, a specialist in the psychology of eating, focuses on the metabolic power of pleasure and relaxation. He tells us, "When you're turned on by food, you turn on your metabolism." Marc shares the knowledge we've gained in study after study and arrives at the inescapable conclusion that when we remove pleasure from our dining experiences, the nutritional value of our food plummets.

Long ago I learned that Americans are copycats. And in a similar vein, they like to be told what to do. When I practiced nutrition in Atlanta I ate lunch almost every day at a great little place called Veggieland. I recommended it highly to many of my clients, and often I would run into them there.

One day I noticed that a client of mine was asking Happy, the owner (who was very happy), exactly what I'd ordered. "I want what Carol's having," she ordered.

Happy laughed and said, "But you don't even know what Carol has ordered or whether you'll like it!"

"Doesn't matter—I'll have what she's having."

For a moment I felt like a brunette Sally Albright (Meg Ryan) in *When Harry Met Sally.* Clearly my client presumed that because I was a nutritional consultant I knew something she didn't know, or perhaps there was some special magic in the combination of foods I had ordered. At our next consultation I explained that defining one's own taste and eating style is the end game.

SALLY ALBRIGHT

But I'd like the pie heated and I don't want the ice cream on top, I want it on the side, and I'd like strawberry instead of vanilla if you have it, if not then no ice cream just whipped cream but only if it's real; if it's out of the can then nothing.

WAITRESS

Not even the pie?

SALLY ALBRIGHT

No, I want the pie, but then not heated.

Being that demanding is hard for a lot of people, but that's what it's going to take to enjoy the freedom to be you. It's important to know how you like your eggs and your pie. It's important to honor your family traditions and culture. And it's essential to a healthy metabolism that you find pleasure, authenticity, and honesty in your choices.

To Each Her Own

Speaking of knowing your own mind, allow me to share a short story that goes to show how easy it is to "lose your mind."

Crazy as I know it sounds, when we first moved to New York I slept a little better just knowing there was a nice little French bakery a stone's throw from our apartment. I really didn't frequent the tiny patisserie that often—I just enjoyed knowing it was there. One day, while my husband was out of town on business, I stopped in for a little something sweet. Not quite certain of my mood, I browsed the pastry case a little longer than usual and then finally decided.

"I'll have the French cookie," I said, approaching the cashier.

"After twenty minutes looking, *that's* what you came up with?" the cashier quipped.

"Why?" I asked. "What's wrong with the French cookie?"

"It's dry," she answered, "and it's the most boring thing in the case! I'm starving, and even I don't want it." (You gotta love the New York drama.)

"Okay, then, what would you suggest?" I asked, playing along.

"The strawberry napoleon," she answered without glancing up. "It's creamy and *good*—the strawberries are fresh."

"All right, give me the strawberry napoleon. I like cream," I conceded. And off I went. The napoleon was good and creamy, and the berries were very fresh.

A few days later, when my husband returned from his Sunday bagel run, he surprised me with a little treat from the French bakery—the French cookie.

"I know how much you like that kind of thing," he beamed.

And guess what? To me, and maybe only me, it was delicious—not good but scrumptious. Not at all dry but crumbly—deliciously moist crumbs, just like a delicate crumb cake, another one of my all-time favorites.

Lesson learned. No one knows what's better for me than me—except for this time, maybe my husband! Remember, it doesn't matter what anyone else likes or dislikes. It's all about what *you* crave. You know the old saying: "There's no accounting for taste." Just be sure that you respect your culinary cravings by indulging them once in a while.

Good to the Last Drop

My parents brought me up on the ritual of coffee and conversation. I adore the taste, sound, and aroma of good, strong coffee brewed in a percolator. Lucky for me, I own a nifty Cuisinart electric percolator that, in my opinion, makes the very best coffee. (In fact, I own several; in case they decide to discontinue the model, I keep a few in reserve.) The shiny, stylish retro pot, with a glass bubble in the middle of the lid, indulges my memories. The *blub-blub* of the bubbling coffee is the only wake-up call I need.

A few years ago, at the end of a visit to the West Coast, my husband and I grabbed coffee to go in the San Francisco airport. From that day forward Peet's coffee was our brand of choice. For a while, we had the whole beans delivered at home until finally our local grocer started to stock Peet's. We enjoy the robust, bold flavor of French roast. I grind a bag or two at the supermarket once a week or so.

One morning, "What's wrong with this coffee?" my husband gasped in displeasure after his first sip.

"I don't know," I replied, scratching my head while tasting the wretched brew, until I remembered our last visit to the coffee grinder. "Don't you *remember*?" I asked my husband, with the intensity of a crime scene investigator. "Remember . . . we ground the coffee and our bag overflowed? I think someone left some of their coffee in the machine and tainted ours!"

"Well, it's awful," my husband whined, "just awful. It tastes *flavored*—like chocolate almond."

It *was* awful. But neither of us are wasteful, so we decided to try to use up the coffee we'd brewed. We drank a cup or two and then washed the rest down the drain.

The next day my husband was traveling, so I endured another pot made from the tainted beans and one after that, laced though it was with the fake chocolate almond taste. "Coffee is expensive," I rationalized. "And there are people living with much worse, so I'll buck up and finish the ruined stash."

That weekend, Sunday to be exact, I brewed the bastardized coffee and made our favorite breakfast of fluffy banana pancakes sprinkled with powdered sugar and walnuts and served alongside sunny-side-up eggs. On that morning, against the backdrop of the delicious pancakes, I just couldn't stomach one more drop. I got up, yanked the cord out of the socket, snapped the lid off the percolator, and threw the contents down the drain. I headed to the pantry and tossed the remaining ground coffee into the garbage can.

Popping open a new bag, I took a deep whiff of unadulterated French roast and, upon inhaling the delicious aroma, asked myself, "What the heck were you thinking? You hypocrite, you! You're writing a book about raising the bar, enjoying the best foods available, and not settling for imitation anything." Then and there I snapped out of it, saying to myself, "My body is not a garbage dump, and I am not doing anything to ease world hunger by drinking distasteful coffee."

In that moment of clarity, the value of savoring and respecting my food choices became even more deeply ingrained in me, and that value has shaped my now steadfast philosophy. As you, too, begin to integrate these values into your worldview, you will find that consuming only the best is a natural and fitting way not only to manage your weight but, more important, to nurture your soul.

PRACTICING YOUR FRENCH

This week:

1. If you normally eat breakfast in five minutes, make it ten minutes. Do the same with lunch and dinner. If you normally eat in twenty minutes, make it thirty.
2. Put your fork down between each bite. *Taste and enjoy* the food.
3. Take pleasure in eating your favorite food without naming it good or bad.
4. Prepare eggs just the way you like them.

Interlude
Le Fromage

"How can one be expected to govern a country with two hundred and forty six cheeses?" Charles de Gaulle once asked.

The French woman's position on cheese is no different than her thoughts on anything else in her life. It must be authentic and of high quality. Along with wine, cheese is a central element of a French meal, and an essential item in a French kitchen is a wonderful cheese ripening on a plate. Available in a wide variety of textures, shapes, and flavors, French cheeses are easily categorized by the strength of their flavor.

Mild Flavor

Mild-flavored French cheese is usually paired with a fruity red wine. One of the best-known mild cheeses is *Brie*, popular for its creamy mellowness. *Brillat-Savarin* is decadently delicious, with a buttery flavor and a smooth texture. *Emmental* is slightly sharp and salty, with a harder texture. Although *Cantal* is often aged for stronger flavor, a young *Cantal* cheese is sweet and slightly tangy.

Medium Flavor

Medium-flavored French cheeses are generally served with champagne or a crisp white wine. *Camembert* offers a slightly stronger flavor than Brie, but it has the same buttery texture. Slightly sour and salty, *Chaource* is generally preferred aged. *Mimolette* has a sharp taste with hints of nuts and fruit. Distinctive for its woodsy flavor, *Mont d'Or* is thick and creamy, with a strong aroma, and is best served warm. Crumbly, soft, and tangy, *Neufchâtel* is one of France's oldest cheeses, dating back to the sixth century.

Strong Flavor

Stronger-flavored French cheeses go well with a variety of white and red wines. *Beaufort* offers a sharp taste yet is slightly rich and creamy in texture. *Comté* has strong, complex flavors that include hints of chocolate, butter, apricot, and toast. The uncooked cheese called *Morbier* is both savory and fruity and has a strong aroma. *Saint Marcellin* is creamy, with a light, acidic, somewhat nutty taste. The very smooth-textured *Tomme de Savoie* matures over several months and has a fruity, grassy taste. *Crottin* is a hard goat's milk cheese that has a sharp flavor when aged.

Bold Flavor

Bold French cheeses are often paired with dessert wines or beer. A rich cheese with meaty and nutty flavors, *Munster* is one of the most popular because of its highly aromatic rind. *Bleu d'Auvergne* also has a pungent aroma and a salty, spicy taste. *Fourme d'Ambert* is a creamy blue cheese with tastes of fruit and wine.

Where to buy cheese in Paris? Androuet is a group of shops run by a family that has been producing and selling some of the best cheeses France has to offer for more than 100 years. Part of the secret of their success is that the owners base their family's reputation on the cheese they sell, so they make sure that the quality of their wares is never compromised.

Here are the addresses of the seven Androuet cheese shops in Paris:

37 rue de Verneuil – 75007 Paris
17 rue des Belles-Feuilles – 75016 Paris
23 rue de la Terrasse – 75017 Paris
134 rue Mouffetard – 75005 Paris
1 rue Bois le Vent – 75016 Paris
93 rue de Cambronne – 75015 Paris
Aéroport Charles de Gaulle Halls 2E et S3 – Paris Roissy – Airport

The stores attract a loyal local clientele as well as travelers from around the world who will be happy to know that a recent expansion initiative means there are now boutique Androuet shops throughout Europe. To locate one, visit http://androuet. com/cheese-shop.html. ✿

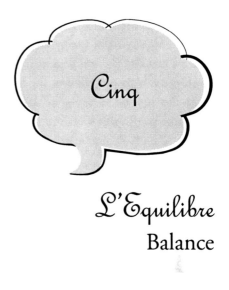

Cinq

L'Equilibre
Balance

Everything in moderation, including moderation.

—*Julia Child*

THE FIFTH SECRET of the French woman—maintaining a balance between stress and pleasure, between indulging in wonderful food and burning calories—may be the most subjective of all because it means managing and coordinating all the aspects of your busy life.

My client Blanche runs a very successful business but is on the road quite a bit and deals with a fair amount of stress in her job. She has struggled with her weight most of her life, beginning when her mother wrapped her in a girdle at some point in her early teens. Her mother examined every bite she took. When she got married, her husband declared that he would rather that she have cancer than remain overweight. (Yes, he is now her ex-husband.)

Overweight and happily divorced, Blanche met a great guy, the man of her dreams. Her new husband provides her with unconditional love and support, so she decided to take her weight management into her own hands.

From One Extreme . . .

Blanche met with "a weight-loss specialist" and existed on a daily regimen of 10 ounces of protein and sparse servings of vegetables. In a year she lost 100 pounds. When I met her, she was beginning to gain weight and was on a vegan diet.

On the high-protein diet she had been constantly constipated, so a high-fiber vegan diet seemed to be a good idea. Not to mention that so many people said you could lose weight this way. And more than anything, she wanted to "taste" again; she couldn't even look at another chicken breast.

Embarked on a new plan, Blanche found a vegan restaurant some thirty miles away where she indulged several times a week in seemingly safe choices like tasty pumpkin squash soup and a variety of vegetable dishes. It wasn't until she complained to the owner that she was gaining weight that he informed her of the high calorie content of her favorites—for example, his delicious and flavorful soups were laced with rich coconut milk. Also, when pressed she admitted that since she automatically deemed the vegan dishes healthy, she ate whatever she wanted and as much as she wanted.

Meanwhile, Blanche's intestines, having been denied fiber for so long, reacted to the vegan diet with shock and entered a state of intense activity. During our first meeting she made several emergency trips to the ladies' room.

Two dieting extremes were in play for Blanche, but where, oh where, was the balance? Protein is a good idea, and so are vegetables, and certainly the food Blanche was eating on the vegan diet was healthy. One idea I suggested was for her to look at the value of each program and extract the best of each, while considering all of her personal factors (extensive business travel, dining out in a different city every day, no time for cooking) until she achieved a hybrid style of eating tailored just for her.

It sounds simple, doesn't it, and, truly, that's our goal: that weight management be simple—and balanced.

But finding equilibrium doesn't happen overnight, particularly if you've been out of whack for some time. Personally, my method has been to replace my obsession with food restrictions with an obsession with balance.

Recently my left index finger was aching. I know that the discomfort is the result of an inflammatory issue—as much as I hate to admit it, possibly a little arthritis. My inner wisdom was whispering, "A few dietary changes may help—less sugar, more foods with omega fatty acids."

At the same time, I dug in my heels, remembering all of the days of deprivation, of eating solely for health, with no regard for pleasure. "I love the freedom of eating what suits me. I don't want to go back to that place of rules and restrictions." I ran the words over and over in my mind.

As the scales of balance swung to the left, then back to the right, my mind followed every shift, every feeling, until I was finally able to achieve the steady, horizontal place in the center, stabilizing the scales.

In place of a screeching U-turn in the road, I opted for moderation—a little less sugar, a little more oily fish, and some physical therapy in the form of hand and finger exercises. Without much thought, sacrifice, effort, or drama, the discomfort subsided naturally in no time at all.

. . . To Another

Ironically, a couple of months later I received a call from Blanche. "I've lost thirty-five pounds," she squealed.

"Terrific," I responded enthusiastically, assuming she had followed my advice.

"Well, you won't be happy with the way I did it," she confessed. "I went to a doctor and started the HCG diet. Besides the injections, the low-calorie plan was just what I needed—I just had to divorce myself from food. I have to accept it: I can never eat carbs again."

My heart sank. I couldn't find the words to express myself at length to Blanche at that moment, so I simply said, "Well, Blanche, never say never." Blanche knows, and you know, that I do not endorse quick fixes or fad diets in general. In this case, because of the absurdity associated with HCG, I owe you a particular warning.

HCG (human chorionic gonadotropin) is a hormone produced during pregnancy by the cells that form the placenta. While it is most commonly associated with pregnancy, it is present in both genders. HCG signals the hypothalamus (the area of the brain that affects metabolism) to break down ingested fats into simpler compounds that can be used by the cells of the body. In pregnancy, this helps the body bring nutrients into the placenta, fueling the fetus with the energy to grow. The HCG diet—a daily ration of 500 calories plus injections of the hormone—promises to help you lose from 1 to 3 pounds per day.

Eating only 500 calories per day is severely restrictive. During the Holocaust, prisoners were given 900–1,000 calories daily while they were held captive in concentration camps.

In fact, 500 calories per day are not enough to support normal brain function. Your body will compensate by using stores of glycogen (stored carbohydrates), protein (muscle), and some fat, which in fact *lowers* your resting metabolism. You may lose weight initially, but you won't be able to keep it off. The body is a pretty efficient machine, and in an effort to save your life, it will react to starvation mode by shutting down and converting whatever little food you do consume into fat.

Then there's the question of how long you can stand to be on such a diet, and in the meantime you will be so irritable, lightheaded, and cranky that at any given moment you'll be at risk of snapping, reaching for whatever food you can get your hands on, and having a field day. Let's just say for the sake of argument that you manage to grin and bear the wacky diet. Is the weight loss sustainable?

Sustainable weight loss is achieved through sensible, balanced eating and moderate exercise based on our individual daily requirements. Our bodies (specifically, our metabolisms) are not designed for the on-again, off-again, abusive behavior of caloric restriction and subsequent bingeing. We cannot outsmart the wisdom of our bodies. As long as we continue starving and bingeing and not expending the calories we consume in a recurring way, we leave the body with no alternative but to pile up the unburned food reserves, leading to the endless cycle of weight gain, weight loss, weight gain, weight loss.

Plus, with HCG, there's the fact that you may feel like you're pregnant—swelling, breast tenderness, and water retention sound good to you? More serious and life-threatening side effects, including an increased risk of blood clots, headaches, restlessness, and depression, have been associated with the use of HCG. Not the least of these is a potentially life-threatening condition called ovarian hyperstimulation syndrome (OHSS).

There is no scientific evidence supporting HCG injections as a weight-loss strategy.* In addition, these injections have not been approved by the FDA for use in weight loss. In fact, since 1975 the FDA has required all marketing and advertising of HCG to state the following: "HCG has not been demonstrated to be effective adjunctive therapy in the treatment of obesity. There is no substantial evidence that it increases weight loss beyond that resulting from calorie restriction, that it causes a more attractive or 'normal' distribution of fat, or that it decreases the hunger and discomfort associated with calorie-restricted diets."

Blanche's unwise choice of the HCG diet is but one example. There have been many absurd miracle cures before this one, including, in the 1800s, a scheme involving the ingestion of a tapeworm. (I did not make that up.) Beyond the fact that they don't work in the long run, these gimmicks keep people from taking sensible and effective steps to do the only thing that does work for successful weight management: change their eating habits.

The Stress Factor

Gabrielle booked an appointment with me based on a referral from a friend. I was excited to have her as a client. I knew her casually—she owned and operated a lovely shop in town and was clearly very creative and talented, not to mention a successful entrepreneur.

I find it interesting that so many of my clients excel in their professional lives yet struggle to manage their weight. On the surface it would seem that the same type of discipline would apply to both. Yet clearly emotional issues muddy the water when it comes to weight management.

Because of her hectic schedule, my first meeting with Gabrielle was after normal business hours. A single parent of two teenage boys, Gabrielle is a very involved parent who races back and forth between football practice and other after-school activities while managing her shop and traveling on buying trips—all the things managing a business and a family entails.

After she completed the client questionnaire, we sat down to talk. Typically I ask a few health and lifestyle questions and move into some preliminary suggestions and a strategy for the next session. In this case we never moved on.

Once Gabrielle started venting, she never stopped. Not for more than ninety minutes. I was flattered that she felt safe sharing her frustrations and concerns with me. I listened intently as she spoke rapidly, almost breathlessly, while remaining quite ladylike, as only a true Southerner can pull off. Gabrielle was animated and funny, but underneath her beautiful blonde facade she was as stressed-out as anyone I had ever met.

I believed her when she said that she wasn't eating much. God knows, she didn't have the time. And she exercised regularly—which, given her stress level, was a very good thing. Yet there she sat, caught up in a never-ending battle of stress, dieting, hunger, weight gain, and more stress.

As I analyzed Gabrielle's body type, I noticed that almost all of her excess weight was belly fat. Given her description of her eating habits and her demanding schedule, this made sense to me. Also, as she talked, I had observed the veins in her forehead bulging (a sign of stress), leaving no doubt in my mind that cortisol, the hormone that accounts for belly fat, was pumping though her system in record amounts.

Here's the thumbnail account of cortisol as it relates to body fat and our health: Where we store fat has everything to do with stress. Heightened levels of stress are associated with greater levels of abdominal fat.* And compared with fat stored in other parts of the body, belly fat is linked with serious health risks such as heart disease.

Here's a slightly more detailed version: A hormone produced by the adrenal glands, cortisol helps regulate blood pressure and cardiovascular function, as well as the body's use of proteins, carbohydrates, and fats. It is often called a "stress hormone" because the secretion of cortisol increases in response to chronic physical and psychological stress. An increased cortisol level is linked to added belly fat because an enzyme that controls cortisol production is present in heavy concentrations in abdominal fat, both visceral (internal fat that accumulates among the organs) and subcutaneous (the more superficial fat immediately under the skin).

So cortisol has an effect on weight management. Most directly, too much stress (and cortisol) can slow your metabolism and set the stage for weight gain. And prolonged stress can affect your blood sugar levels and the mood swings and fatigue that go with them. Chronic stress and associated higher cortisol levels have even been linked to metabolic syndrome, a group of health concerns that can lead to serious problems like heart attacks and diabetes.*

The rubber meets the road at the intersection of stress and emotional eating. When you're stressed, you may find dieting difficult, and you are more likely to go for the junk food since cravings for fatty, salty, and sugary foods are more prevalent when people are experiencing chronic stress. High levels of cortisol not only make you yearn for unhealthy food; nervous energy also can lead you to devour anything that distracts you from the stressful situation at hand.

"The term 'dieting' brings to mind deprivation, starvation, being miserable and uncomfortable and ultimately failing in weight loss efforts," says Samantha Heller, a dietitian, nutritionist, and exercise physiologist,* noting that burning more calories than you consume is how your body loses weight. "However, severe calorie restriction, diet fads, pills and potions, detox cleanses and other quacky approaches to weight loss only contribute to people's diet failures and, in fact, may increase the likelihood of regaining even more weight than what was lost—if any," Heller adds, reinforcing the negative impact of stress. "The best way to drop unwanted pounds is to adopt healthy lifestyle behaviors that include eating a variety of quality foods, physical activity, patience, and a game plan," she says.

Dr. David L. Katz, director of the Prevention Research Center at Yale University School of Medicine, chimes in to explain that there are ways to help reduce stress on the way to a healthier lifestyle. In general, dieting alone is not all that useful, he says. "Eating well and being active for life is the way to go. Food itself, a reliable source of immediate gratification, may be used to relieve stress.

When food intake is restricted, something else should replace it." Dr. Katz goes on to report that in consuming more nutritional foods you can be satisfied by fewer calories, without deprivation.

I wish I could tell you that Gabrielle's stress has lessened. However, as with a lot of us, her proverbial plate is still quite full. We've become dear friends since meeting for that first consultation, so I know that she has traveled several times to Paris, which has become one of her favorite destinations—an escape from her day-to-day challenges. Recently she emailed me from there: "Why on earth did I choose a hotel right across the street from the best patisserie in Paris?"

I answered, "Because you are meant to spend quality time with yourself, slipping right into that patisserie each and every day for a sip of something hot and one perfect macaron in honor of *le goûter.*" If that doesn't fend off the cortisol, I don't know what will.

Looking for Answers in All the Wrong Places

> *Your karma is in the refrigerator.*
> —Donald Altman, *"Art of the Inner Meal"*

"Are the answers in the refrigerator?" I ask my husband.

"What?"

"The answers you're looking for, did you find them in the refrigerator?"

Wearing only boxer shorts and leaning in farther, he answers, "No, I actually found them in the freezer," as he removes the frozen coconut cake from its box.

Uh oh . . . that cake is history, yet another victim of Sunday night, back to work Monday morning apprehension.

"Starving all day and on the prowl all night" is how another client, a prominent local professional, described his eating regimen. In his working life, he interacts with people under very exacting conditions, and the result used to be a free-for-all once he was back in the safety of his own home—more specifically, his own kitchen.

This is not at all what we expect from men, whom we tend to view as less emotionally driven than women. Perhaps, for anyone, emotional eating is simply a result of the discomfort of unwanted feelings. Men and women alike tend to want to avoid painful feelings; we could say they *swallow* them as they overindulge in food—a way to stuff their emotions down to a place where they can be ignored for a while.

Additionally, eating becomes a way to disassociate from thoughts and feelings that make us uncomfortable. It is a temporary distraction from the products of our restless minds. But notice the word "temporary." When the cake is gone, the feeling, the issue, the conflict, or the problem is still very much present—along with the additional pounds.

Reams of material have been written about emotional eating, and we can analyze our actions until the cows come home. But the bottom line is that many of us have gotten ourselves into an unhealthy habit—one of substituting food for life. We feed our stomach when it is really our soul that needs to be fed.

You and only you know the answer to the question "What is troubling you?" All that is necessary is to sit with the question long enough to let the answer and your feelings surface.

In the case of my client it was really very simple. He was a pretty uptight guy during his working day. When he walked in the door to his wife and children each evening, he breathed a huge sigh of relief; unfortunately, he experienced that relief most fully when he gave free rein to his food cravings.

Eventually he allowed himself the time he needed to look carefully and closely into his behavior. He remembered coming home from school to his mother, waiting for him in the kitchen with an indulgent snack—a reward for the seriousness and diligence he always brought to his studies. His habit of eating for emotional comfort had begun way back when he was a schoolboy striving for stellar grades.

Having made the connection, he enlisted the help of his family. The kids put up "No Prowling" signs in the kitchen. He entered through the front door of his house rather than into the kitchen, where he had become accustomed to making an immediate pit stop at the pantry. His wife continued to serve balanced meals and insisted he wait for the dinner bell.

After dinner he picked up his guitar instead of a bag of chips and headed for the basement to enjoy a much-loved, yet ignored pastime. He was able, with the help of his loving family, to break his bad eating habits. No magic dust, just a good strategy and a loving support group.

The Secret Is Balance

We've heard that French women don't get fat, and of course we know that women are women. French, American—we all share the same desires, but we base our eating habits on different fundamentals. The difference is that the French display an innate *balance*.

A devoted Web surfer, I came across a wonderful article in the online magazine *The Morning News* (themorningnews.org).* Published on March 28, 2005, it was a roundtable discussion conducted by Josh Friedland, who operates a terrific website called The Food Section (thefoodsection.com). Josh had assembled four successful French food bloggers—Pascale Weeks, Clotilde Dusoulier, Estelle Tracy, and Requia Badr—to discuss the French Paradox. Their comments fit so beautifully into *The French Twist* that, with Josh's permission, I'm including them, starting below and every so often hereafter throughout the book.

Here's what French food blogger Pascale Weeks (look for her at www.goosto.fr, a French food site) has to say about maintaining balance in her eating habits:

> I eat chocolate nearly every day, but only a small amount and only a good quality chocolate like Valrhona, for example.
>
> I really enjoy wine and drink some twice a week. On the other hand, I never drink any other alcohol.
>
> I love cheese, but not at the end of a meal as I find it too rich. I eat cheese mostly for lunch with a bowl of soup and a piece of good bread.
>
> Even though I love pastries, I eat them when I have friends for dinner (homemade pastries) or when I go to a restaurant for dinner if I'm sure it's made by the restaurant. I also love croissants, but I have one only once a week. Of course, if I go by Pierre Hermé or Ladurée (among the most famous patisseries in Paris), I might have a *macaron*. I rarely eat pastries which are not homemade and rarely pastries with cream.

Clotilde Dusoulier, a Parisian who lives in Montmartre and who is the author of the blog *Chocolate & Zucchini: Daily Adventures in a Parisian Kitchen*, tells us:

> The secret lies in one word (and a hyphenated one at that): self-discipline. Most of us will allow ourselves a splurge from time to time, but not every day, and we'll try to compensate by eating less the next day and exercising regularly. We will indulge in wine, cheese, and chocolate, but will restrain ourselves (however much we want that extra slice of *tarte tatin*) and stop at a reasonable serving. And when we notice that we've put on a couple pounds or more the panic is optional, but we will cut down on sweets, unnecessary fat, and alcohol until we're back where we feel comfortable. This technique works and seems to be profoundly built into our behavior (we've seen our mothers and friends do it), but I don't think it comes

easy to anyone as it requires daily attention. But then again, who ever said life was an all-you-can-eat buffet?

Balance is vital; fruits, vegetables, protein, and fat play interdependent roles, interacting with each other and with your body processes. Without carbohydrates you can't process protein effectively. If you don't eat protein, your body takes fuel from your own lean muscle, slowing your metabolic rate. Essential fatty acids are a vital component in the production of hormones. If you neglect any category, you won't get adequate supplies of the nutrients you need.

If you consider your body as a furnace, your goal is to have a hot, constant flame. Protein is the wood. Carbohydrates are the starter. If you eat just protein, the flame may never catch. If you eat just carbohydrates, you're going to have a flame that burns hot and then dies out quickly.

PRACTICING YOUR FRENCH

This week:

1. Think about someone you admire when it comes to balanced eating, and replicate their eating practices. List as many of their characteristics as you can. What benefits would you expect if you ate as this person does?

2. Think about how the standards you set for your diet relate to the standards you set for yourself as a person. Are they realistic and balanced?

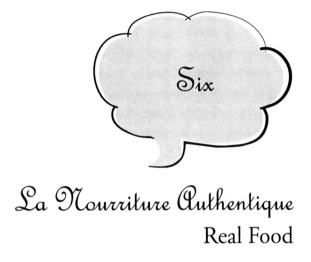

La Nourriture Authentique
Real Food

How can a nation be called great
if its bread tastes like Kleenex?
—Julia Child

I ALWAYS KNEW THE FRENCH were serious about food. But whereas many baby boomers had their first taste of Europe in college, it wasn't until I was in my thirties that I actually experienced the flavor of Europe. My age may have been an advantage, given how much experience and maturity had heightened my appreciation for such inspiring cuisine.

I marveled at all the good food, made from the simplest local and real ingredients, that was served in the smallest bistros. There were no artificial sugar packets on the table or plastic containers of fake cream for coffee. I questioned why things were so different in America. Surely in the land of plenty we have the raw ingredients— world-class beef, abundant fish, and acres of fruits and vegetables. I soon learned that despite all we had, there was something missing in our approach to food: an insistence on fresh, high-quality foods prepared and enjoyed with passion.

My research clarified for me that as we had industrialized as a nation we had moved further and further from the food source and closer and closer to faux foods.

Keeping It Real

In chapter 3, we looked at the secret of favoring quality over quantity, and laid out several categories of quality foods—foods that not only taste good but can make a real difference in our health and our appearance.

Another aspect of quality is authenticity, and keeping it real is the sixth secret. Here in the United States we don't have routine access to the same fresh, authentic, quality foods that the French find all around them. At the same time, the French are not accustomed to the mass marketing and nonstop advertising efforts of American food conglomerates. The marketing of fake foods has, at least in part, contributed to our unfortunate number-one position as the nation with the highest level of obesity in the world.

In France and throughout Europe, food is plucked ripe from the vine, the river, or the farmyard and arrives on a local plate within the day. In the United States, our produce is harvested well before it's ready, thrown into a truck, and hauled halfway across the country. Most cattle, pigs, and chickens live in horrifying confinement that, besides the moral issues involved, creates the perfect scenario for the rapid spread of bacteria and disease.

We have little concern about where our food comes from, particularly if it's been processed with who knows what preservatives in order to assure a long shelf life.

Despite the fact that we Americans are more health-conscious than ever and that we have access to the most cutting-edge nutritional science, severe illnesses—obesity, diabetes, heart disease, cancer, and other chronic maladies—continue to prevail in the United States.

Perhaps disease has much to do with the prevalence of processed and artificial foods. When it comes to our nation's livestock we only need to think back as far as the 1940s, when antibiotics were developed and modified for use in the farming industry. In the United States, almost 50 percent of all antibiotics are administered to farm animals. These drugs form a toxic residue in animal tissue—in other words, in the meat we eat. (That begins to explain, by the way, why every year we experience an increase in the number of salmonella poisoning cases from contaminated eggs, meat, and milk. The many strains of salmonella are difficult to treat because they are resistant to antibiotics.)

In addition, farm animals are fed growth-promoting hormones, appetite stimulants, and all kinds of pesticides, fertilizers, and herbicides that, again, accumulate in the animals' tissues and milk.

And we eat and drink it all without a thought about where it comes from.

Who profits from the way food is produced, marketed, and studied in the United States? Let's consider what the processed-food industry has at risk: Its gross revenues represent 13 percent of the U.S. Gross National Product.* A considerable amount of research and nutritional data comes from or is subsidized by food corporations, and the food industry looks out for its own best interests with intensive lobbying and large campaign contributions to government officials who monitor our food quality and safety. It's a telling commentary on where we are as a society that often our public policies place corporate profits above our health.

In turn, academic nutritionists can influence the federal government's food policy. Yet professional integrity is compromised when food companies help offset the costs of producing academic journals, underwrite professional conferences, sponsor research, and even "purchase" entire academic departments.* All of this leaves me wondering about the probability for dubious activity in the areas of government regulation and consumer awareness.

So who can we trust to tell us what kind of food is good for our health? We trust and value scientific research above all else as the final authority, don't we? We mere mortals certainly do not possess the knowledge and expertise necessary to understand the cutting-edge scientific findings on nutrition. Are we to decide what to inspect and what not to inspect, what to trust and what not to trust? These are the questions I asked myself until I came up with another source of information that, from my point of view, is equally reliable, if not more so:

Experience.

In other words, how did people eat before food systems were industrialized, and how good was their health and longevity? What might we learn from traditional, non-industrialized cultures? Even more relevant to this book, what might we learn from the French?

The French choose their foods and processing methods very differently from the way Americans do, and always have done. They understand that the further a food product is from its natural form the less it retains its healthful nutritional properties. In processed foods, vitamins have evaporated, minerals have leached out, and fiber is long gone—a trade-off the French have never been willing to make.

Regardless of their social background, French people cook at home more than Americans do. Many of us rely more than we'd like to admit on dining out or on take-out, and if pressed, we'd have to admit we're often not sure we're eating food made from quality ingredients.

French food is real food—prepared in the kitchen; in France, time is devoted to deliberate selection of ingredients and careful preparation of meals. Buying fresh

REAL VERSUS FAKE: THE CHOICE IS CLEAR

Open your mouth and close your eyes,
and you will get a big surprise!
——My mom

The whole foods that humans have been eating the longest are the very foods that we're the best adapted for. Let's use butter versus margarine as an example. Humans learned to make butter from milk around 3000 b.c. The butter versus margarine debate has been around pretty much since 1870, when margarine was first created in a lab.

The simple way to market a fake food is to demonize the product you want to replace. The margarine versus butter controversy might be the first example of a fake, industrial food replacing a real food that has been in use in healthy cultures for centuries.

What's in butter? Cream and salt. That was easy.

What's in margarine? Hope you've got a minute: liquid canola oil, water, partially hydrogenated soybean oil, plant stanol esters, salt, emulsifiers (vegetable mono- and diglycerides, soy lecithin), hydrogenated soybean oil, potassium sorbate, citric acid and calcium disodium EDTA to preserve freshness, artificial flavor, DL-alpha-Tocopheryl acetate, and vitamin A palmitate. Oh, and it's colored with beta-carotene.

Make a particular note of the third ingredient in the list above: partially hydrogenated soybean oil—a trans fat. These ingredients come from the label of a product called Benecol—a brand the American Heart Association suggests you use in place of butter. Yes, that's right . . . the AHA is suggesting you *eat trans fats to replace butter!* Is the AHA interested in protecting your heart or their wallet? Note that the group accepts payments from the companies that reap the rewards of your shift from butter to fake food. I rest my case.

produce and whipping up a salad or pasta sauce isn't that big of a deal to the French, no matter how busy they may be.

The bottom line is that home cooking provides better control of food. The home-cooking tradition of the French delivers undeniable nutritional benefits. They understand that the more they do to prepare food from scratch, the better their health will be. Plus they get the added reward of looking and feeling great. And if you eat at home regularly, you are likely to be eating significantly lower levels of preservatives, trans fats, sugar, and salt than your peers who mostly eat meals made in restaurants, delis, or fast-food joints.

The Truth About Processed Foods

In 2010 NBC's Jeff Rossen investigated low-fat and low-calorie frozen meals. These meals are advertised as secret weapons to combat weight loss, and consumers love them. But if Americans are consuming these healthy meals, why can't they lose weight? Well, it's the FDA's fault, Rossen reports.* Under the law, food companies are allowed a variance of 20 percent in stating the fat and calorie content on their food labels.

How dare they preach about obesity and trick us this way! Here are some comments from shoppers who were interviewed on the subject:

"That's actually scary because I eat those a lot—
maybe that's why my weight won't budge."

"That's what I look at—
the calories, even before the price."

"I don't buy it because it tastes good;
I buy it because of the calories."

EMSL, an independent testing laboratory, tested the calorie and fat content in the frozen meals, and the results did not match the labels. The numbers were all over the place: Some actually contained fewer calories than stated, some more; the same goes for the fat content.* Susan Roberts, PhD, a food scientist at Tufts University who has done her own investigative audit, thinks that perhaps this is one explanation why Americans are not losing weight.

Really?

If we consume a meal that we believe is 230 calories and it turns out to be 276 calories—*this* is why American's can't lose weight? Get real—and I mean that literally: *Get real!*

Instead, the problem with frozen dinners more likely stems from the artificial ingredients they contain. I consider any item that does not grow in nature to be artificial, and artificial food is not good for us. When we consume artificial food, we are not only getting less nutritional value than that provided by authentic food; we are also putting ourselves at risk of side effects both known and unknown.

Why do we choose artificial foods over real foods in the first place? In addition to valuing convenience over substance, diet dogma affects our choices.

Take low-fat frozen dinners, for example. Fat makes us fat, right? So low-fat must be good, right? Wrong.

Essential fatty acids are . . . how shall I put it? . . . *essential.* We need to obtain these fats from our diet to avoid malnutrition. Fats slow the absorption of nutrients so that you feel satisfied. Fats aid in sugar and insulin metabolism, which helps you lose weight. Fat is your flavorful, filling friend.

When you buy fat-free or sugar-free foods—which, by the way, are not popular in France—the fat and sugar are replaced with artificial ingredients. Unlike with fat and sugar, we have no idea how consuming these artificial items will affect our long-term health.

Mass production of our food contributes to the list of fake foods. Many of the unrecognizable ingredients on our food labels actually come from natural food sources, like wheat or corn, but are so altered by the time they are added to the food that they contain very few of the nutrients found in the original food source. Additives, preservatives, herbicides, antibiotics, and genetic modification compromise the farm-to-market experience so that what is sold on supermarket shelves is no longer real food. Instead it's mass-produced "food product." Cheez Whiz is *not* real cheese.

Some artificial ingredients are added to processed foods to add back the flavor, nutrients, color, and texture that have been eliminated from the food during processing. The FDA allows flavor enhancers to be referred to as "natural flavor." That term is misleading. A flavor enhancer is, more often than not, a chemical approximation of a known food that has been manufactured in a lab.

Other artificial ingredients—namely, preservatives—are added to prolong the shelf life of food. For example, pre-shredded cheese contains anti-caking agents as well as antibiotics to inhibit mold growth. Our preoccupation with convenience is detrimental to the quality of our food. Why not upgrade from a bag of shredded cheese to a nice wedge of cheese imported from France?

Besides the addition of artificial ingredients, processing can mean substituting cheaper versions or using ingredients that are robbed of their nutritional value and then "enriched." High-fructose corn syrup is making the news these days. Research is beginning to suggest that this liquid sweetener may upset the human metabolism, increasing the risk for heart disease and diabetes. And don't judge a book by its cover. Just because you see a sprinkling of oats on the outside of a loaf of bread does not mean that you are choosing whole grains. Look again, and read labels closely.

If processing and the addition of artificial ingredients were not enough, our food supply is becoming heavily affected by genetic modification, the process of permanently combining genetic material from genetically unrelated organisms. The results are new foods such as super pigs with human growth genes, fish with cow growth genes, tomatoes with fish genes, and thousands of other combinations. These creations—genetically modified organisms, or GMOs— are being patented, sold, consumed, and released into the environment, often with little fanfare and, worse, sometimes without even being labeled as genetic modifications.

Currently, up to 45 percent of U.S. corn is genetically engineered, as are 85 percent of our soybeans. The Center for Food Safety has estimated that 70 to 75 percent of processed foods on supermarket shelves—from soda to soup, crackers to condiments—contains genetically engineered ingredients.

We have no information on the long-term health consequences of consuming GMO food. And on a broader ecological scale, the widespread use of GMO products may be threatening the extinction of many original species of plants and animals.

The Great Pretenders

A processed food is any food that has been canned, frozen, or dehydrated or that has had chemicals added to prolong shelf life, provide texture, or enhance taste. Now that you've read that definition, get ready for what may be a startling statistic: Processed foods account for 60 percent of the American diet, in the form of refined grains, vegetable oils, and added sugars.

Here's more on some of the major offenders that go into the great pretenders:

Trans Fatty Acids

The addition of these artificial, hydrogenated oils containing high levels of trans fats allows convenience foods like cookies, chips, crackers, baked goods, and bread to sit on the shelf for months while still retaining their "freshness." I realize this makes absolutely no sense, but that is the claim. A *New England Journal of Medicine* review of more than eighty studies found that trans fats are more dangerous to health than any food contaminant, even when they constitute only 1–3 percent of total calorie intake. The study also showed that you need to eat only 20–60 calories from artificial trans fats a day to damage your health.* And just a 2 percent increase in trans fatty acids in the diet increases the chance of heart disease by 23 percent.

Refined Grains

Refined grains are good grains gone bad. White rice and white flour have had both the bran (the fiber-rich outer layer) and the nutrient-rich germ removed from the grain. Although vitamins and minerals are added back into refined grains after the milling process (this is called "enriching"), they don't end up with as many nutrients as whole grains; in particular, they have less iron and natural fiber.

Why in the world go through the trouble to refine grains? Simply leave the grain be and we're good to go—right? That would be correct, except that someone needs to make a little dough (no pun intended) on the deal. Corporations benefit financially when they can refine the grains, use the bran and germ for other purposes (such as animal feed), and stretch the now-depleted grains by adding fats, chemicals, sugar, and salt.

A slice of supermarket white bread has 66 calories, 1.9 grams of protein, and 0.6 grams of fiber, whereas the same supermarket offers whole-wheat bread, and that slice has 69 calories and provides 3.6 grams of protein and 1.9 grams of fiber. Which would you rather eat?

Buyer beware. Foods "made with wheat flour" or promoted as "seven grain" could very well be the same old refined stuff with a few add-ons—the same stuff that raises the risk for high cholesterol, high blood pressure, heart attacks, insulin resistance, diabetes, and belly fat. When you choose whole grains over refined grains such as white bread, rolls, sugary low-fiber cereal, white rice, or white pasta, you can lower your heart attack risk by up to 30 percent. Plus, high-fiber foods make you feel full longer.

High-Fructose Corn Syrup

You might not know HFCS is there, especially if your palate has adjusted to the unnecessary sugary taste it lends to many frozen foods, or the appealing brown color and soft texture it adds to whole-wheat bread, hamburger buns, and English muffins. We might expect it in soft drinks—they're supposed to be sweet—but it's also added to beer, bacon, spaghetti sauce, and even ketchup. We each consume, on average, nearly 63 pounds of this sneaky syrup per year in artificial food products.

HFCS has found its way into just about everything on the supermarket shelf because it's cheap and sweet. Processed versions of peanut butter, baking mixes, jams and jellies—you name it—all rely on HFCS to enhance flavors, but unfortunately they also include extra calories because of the addition of unnecessary sugar, the last thing we need. While our consumption of refined sugar has slowly dwindled in the past forty years, our consumption of HFCS has shot up almost twenty-fold.

Tufts University researchers reported that Americans consume more calories from HFCS than from any other source, while the French continue to eat modest amounts of table sugar (sucrose). Here we go again: The French choose the real thing. They know what a food's taste should be—as nature intended it. The artificial sugary taste of HFCS that is used to "enhance" food does not appeal to them. Instead, when they need to sweeten their coffee or berries they use good old sugar . . . just a sprinkle to develop the natural taste. And by doing so, they naturally consume fewer calories.

Some researchers say that HFCS's chemical structure encourages overeating. From a physiological perspective it seems to force the liver to pump more heart-threatening triglycerides into the bloodstream. In addition, fructose may zap your body's reserves of chromium, a mineral important for healthy levels of cholesterol, insulin, and, last but not least, the regulation of blood sugar, which could partly explain the overeating that is associated with consumption of high-fructose corn syrup.

A study done at the University of Pennsylvania found that fructose doesn't suppress levels of the hunger hormone ghrelin the way that glucose does. Women who ate fructose instead of glucose had higher ghrelin levels throughout the day, overnight, and into the next day. Bottom line: If you eat or drink HFCS, you'll actually continue to want to consume more calories, even twenty-four hours later, than you would have had you eaten plain table sugar.

Glutamates

What in the world are glutamates? Don't think you eat them? Well, if you've eaten Doritos or ranch dressing, Cheetos, Campbell's soup, Lipton instant soup, Planter's salted nuts, or even the grilled chicken filet at McDonald's, you most certainly have.

The big name in glutamates is monosodium glutamate (MSG), a flavor enhancer first introduced in this country more than fifty years ago. Heralded as a miracle food enhancer, it suppressed bitterness, improved flavor, made food smell better, and removed the tinny taste from canned products. There was even talk that it could improve a person's IQ.

American food manufacturers quickly embraced MSG and began adding it to all kinds of foods, including salad dressings, tuna fish, sausages, and frozen dinners. Before long, restaurants were using it regularly, as were meal programs at airlines, schools, and military bases. Even consumers got into the act, sprinkling MSG, under the brand name Accent, on dishes that needed a little punch.

As MSG became more widely used in the United States, reports began to surface about negative reactions to it. In 1968 the *New England Journal of Medicine* printed a letter from a doctor who experienced numbness at the back of his neck, general weakness, and heart palpitations after eating foods containing MSG. Others complained about headaches, nausea, dizziness, disorientation, and depression.

Despite heaps of evidence, MSG sensitivity remains unacknowledged by many in the food industry and the government. To make matters worse, some labels are being altered to hide the fact that products contain MSG. A few companies have gone so far as to advertise "No MSG" when their products actually contain the substance. The Food and Drug Administration (FDA) has even listed MSG as one of the safest food additives, along with vinegar and salt.

Research shows that MSG acts as a drug, inducing nerve-cell discharges to create a heightened taste sensation. For this reason, it has been classified as an excitatory neurotoxin (excitotoxin, for short), similar to aspartame (NutraSweet). Therefore, many people who react negatively to MSG also cannot tolerate aspartame.*

Artificial Sweeteners

Researchers from Purdue University have laboratory evidence that the widespread use of no-calorie sweeteners may actually make it harder for people to control their food intake and thus their body weight.

In one experiment using rats, the researchers compared the consumption of yogurt sweetened with glucose (sugar) and yogurt sweetened with zero-calorie saccharin. They found that the rats eating the artificial sweetener consumed more calories, gained more weight, put on more body fat, and didn't make up for it by cutting back later.

How can that be? Researchers Susan Swithers and Terry Davidson surmised that by breaking the connection between a sweet sensation and high-calorie food, the use of saccharin changes the body's ability to regulate intake.

The idea is that normally when we eat sugar, our body registers sweetness, and very sweet things have lots of calories. We eat the cake, feel satisfied, and stop eating. But when we repeatedly consume diet products this understanding breaks down—there's sweetness, but no calories. As a result, we misjudge the sweetness/calorie relationship in everything we eat and thus may take in too many calories. Meanwhile, people who eat real sugar maintain the awareness of how many calories they are taking in and thus are more likely to self-regulate and naturally eat less.

"The data clearly indicate that consuming a food sweetened with no-calorie saccharin can lead to greater body-weight gain and adiposity than would consuming the same food sweetened with a higher-calorie sugar," the study, published in *Behavioral Neuroscience*, noted.*

Another study, this one at the University of Alberta, Canada, found that baby rats that ate more diet foods in their early years had a greater chance of becoming obese later in life. The researchers call it a "taste-conditioning process." Transferring this to the human realm, I suspect we've been deprived of true sweetness and are not getting mad—just getting even by overdoing it.*

The authors acknowledge that this outcome may not be seen as welcome news by health-care practitioners, who have long recommended low- or no-calorie sweeteners. But they note that their findings match emerging evidence that people who drink more diet drinks are at higher risk for obesity and metabolic syndrome.

Artificial sweeteners in the form of saccharine, aspartame, sucralose, and acesulfame K, which also taste sweet but do not predict the delivery of calories—could have similar effects, say the researchers.

Chemical Additives

The chemicals added to our food in the form of artificial preservatives are intended to prevent spoilage and food poisoning. But it turns out that the artificial preservatives in our food supply age us and cause all kinds of autoimmune diseases, from multiple sclerosis to cancer.

A common preservative, butylated hydroxyanisole (BHA), has been both "generally recognized as safe" by the FDA, while still being "reasonably anticipated to be a human carcinogen." I know, I know, I'm scratching my head too. BHA abounds—in cereal, baked goods, butter, potato chips, sausage, beer, and meat products.

Speaking of meat products, the sodium nitrate in bacon, ham, lunch meat, and hot dogs may give the meat a nice pink color, but after analyzing more than seven thousand studies on diet and cancer risk, the American Institute for Cancer Research estimated that for every 3.5 ounces of processed meat you eat each day (the equivalent of one hot dog and two slices of smoked turkey breast) your risk of colon cancer shoots up by 42 percent.

A recent double-blind, placebo-controlled study in *The Lancet* proved that after preschoolers and grade-school kids ate an additive free-diet for six weeks, then had "safe additives" reintroduced into their diet, hyperactivity levels rose dramatically.* Why is it that we continue to experiment with the health of our children?

Aucunes Fausses Nourritures: No Faux Foods

> *As for butter versus margarine,*
> *I trust cows more than chemists.*
>
> —Joan Gussow, food policy expert

The European Union has tried a couple of times to introduce FDA-style labels showing a standard nutritional calculus on food packaging. But they can't get it done because there's just no interest in it. No one wants or needs it because Europeans are not agonizing over the grams of protein, fat, and carbohydrates in their foods.

The French don't go to the store to buy grams of this or that. They go to buy food.

Years ago my friend Isabelle loved the low-cal drink Tab and shared it with me. I thought it tasted just awful and fake. She said, "If you drink it long enough you'll get to like it."

I asked, "But why—why would I want to try to like it?" Even though I was only twelve years old, I had the sense to know better. Unfortunately, I didn't get smarter with age, and as I got older I tried all of the artificial sweeteners and fake foods.

Garbage always smells like garbage at first, but if you keep sniffing long enough, it becomes tolerable. After a while you may even think it is pleasant.

My friend Colette drinks "cream" with her coffee. When she spent the night with us while traveling from the West Coast, I apologized when I realized we had only milk in the refrigerator to offer her.

"No problem," she chirped. "I have my own." She ran into the guest room and returned with a canister of Coffee-mate flavored with something artificial. My guilt subsided. Quickly.

"Usually I don't drink the stuff from the canister. At home I have the liquid stuff with almond flavoring," Colette said.

"Oh, that's *much* better," I responded sarcastically. Ironically, at the time we were discussing my book and faux foods specifically.

It's not that Colette doesn't know that this cream in a canister is artificial—it's a habit, a bad one that she just doesn't consider as having much to do with thwarting her weight-loss efforts. But the reality is that this artificial food fails to satisfy her healthy and natural fat cravings and does nothing more than set her up to respond unthinkingly and to eat in an excessive way later in the day.

Real will always be better than fake—always. And fake will never be health supportive—never.

Your body does not recognize fake; it can only metabolize that which it can identify—real, whole foods. So enjoy the cream in your morning coffee, and give your taste buds a break. The French will be the first to tell you—simple pleasures never killed anyone, but lack of them can.

There's a good reason why the frozen food and prepared food section of the supermarkets in France is minimal: The French do not purchase prepared, packaged, or frozen foods. The cereals offered in an American supermarket often occupy an entire aisle; in France there are just a few selections, predominantly muesli and other healthy and whole options.

Do you want to know if tilapia is sustainably fished or whether maltodextrin is a harmful additive? Download the apps discussed in the online article "iPhone Apps for Eating Clean and Healthy" on wellsphere.com (http://www.wellsphere.com/parenting-article/iphone-apps-for-eating-clean-and-healthy/1180766) and let your phone guide you through the maze of grocery store do's and don'ts.

Clotilde Dusoulier weighs in on faux foods: "There are a lot of things I just won't eat because they're too processed and full of preservatives and nasty, and I'm just not interested in them. I like things to be fresh and tasty and carefully prepared, so that keeps me away from a lot of things that wouldn't be very good for me."

Estelle Tracy, a native of France who once lived in the suburbs of Paris but now resides near Philadelphia, publishes the blog *Le Hamburger et le Croissant*. She notes, "Almost everything I eat is home-made. We buy a box of Oreo cookies once a year at most, that's it! Processed food is usually less satisfying than homemade, so I try to cook and bake as much as I can. If I don't have enough time to cook, I always have some pasta and a good tomato sauce in my pantry."

For me, faux food is like a hollow chocolate Easter bunny—one disappointing bite renders you hungry and searching for something solid and real.

When shopping for packaged foods, if you do not recognize any of the ingredients, either don't buy the product or educate yourself about the ingredient before buying it. In the meantime, try experimenting with the basics. Eat real, whole foods—and you won't even have to read the label.

Farmers' Markets: Getting Closer to the Source

Markets where farmers offer fresh produce and other products have been around for generations, but it is only within the last decade or so that farmers' markets in the United States have really caught on. There are now more than 6,000 documented farmers' markets in the U.S., and more are opening with each harvest. And it's no wonder—shopping at a farmers' market is a truly enjoyable way to get top-quality food and to connect it with the people who grew it.

The fundamental idea of a farmers' market is that all of the goods available for sale have been produced within a reasonable distance from the market—say, roughly 150 miles. There are no rigid rules; some markets are strictly organic, others sell only produce, and still others combine crafts, prepared foods, houseplants, and even live music with locally produced food.

Within a single market you will find price differences among vendors offering the same crop. Take tomatoes, for example. The farmer who grows organic heirlooms may be charging three times what the non-organic grower is charging. Ask questions. Find out why the prices are different, and buy the best quality you can for your budget.

Cost is the issue many people cite for not shopping at the local farmers' market. While foodies agree, their main argument is that food from a farmers' market is fresher and tastes better than food from a grocery store. I agree that a better product is worth paying more for; however, not everything is more expensive. Because crops become more plentiful as the season progresses, prices tend to go down.

Once you get home, preparing your produce is easy—the simpler the better! Don't overpower the sweetness of summer corn or the juiciness of tomatoes with heavy sauces or seasonings. Eat them raw or lightly cooked. Make salads. Toss pasta with barely sautéed vegetables. Above all, enjoy the gift that is summer, and eat as much seasonal produce as you can.

A good resource for finding farmers' markets in your area is LocalHarvest.org. Visit the site for information about the market and contact details as available.

Why Settle for Stand-Ins?

When I was in the film business, I acted as a stand-in on *Little Man Tate*, Jodi Foster's directorial debut. It sounds exciting, and Jodi Foster *is* the bomb, but even so, it was one of the stranger jobs I ever had in the film business. I was hired in Cincinnati for a shoot in Columbus because I met the Screen Actor's Guild requirements and was the same height, weight, and coloring as Debi Mazar, who played Gina in the film.

Sometimes it can take hours to set up a single shot as the lighting people get their equipment in place and adjusted and the set dressers worry about where to place a prop, along with dozens of other tiny details. Genuine actors like Jodi Foster and Debi Mazar are not expected to have the stamina to wait around while a shot is set up and then is tested in early takes—perhaps dozens of them. Expecting the real actor to provide a fresh performance after enduring all of that prep time just isn't reasonable. This is where the stand-ins come in.

The first thing I did every morning was to head to the wardrobe department to get "color cover" so that I matched Debi. Then a day of "hurry up and wait," until it was time to walk through the scene and stand where I was placed as the shot was composed.

Eventually, the "second team"—that was me—steps out so that the scene can be rehearsed with the "first actors," otherwise known as the "actual actors," playing the roles. Then more waiting. I found it terribly easy to zone out, mainly because a stand-in is a facade rather than a person. I unzipped my head, removed my brain, and set it aside for the day in order to get through the gig.

Stand-in work gets you nowhere. Most of the time you don't even get a credit in the film. It doesn't mean you'll get acting roles—it just means that you happen to be the same size and coloring as the real performer.

It's sort of like faux food—it may look the same on the outside, but it's really just color cover. It won't get you anywhere nutritionally, and it doesn't satisfy you. It won't do a thing for you except keep you waiting for the real deal.

Take, for example, the case of artificial sweeteners standing in for the foods of nature—honey, sugar, and fruit. Artificial sweeteners boast zero calories but zone out when it comes to any nutritional value whatsoever. The pancreas gets a signal to get working and then says, "On what?"

Many years ago I was placing my order at a frozen yogurt counter, and I requested a fat-free, sugar-free yogurt. An older woman standing next to me in line said, "So what's left?" A very good question indeed. What's left? Who knows?

Go ahead—join the second team and unzip your head, remove your brain, set it aside, zone out, and eat fake food.

But wait, there is another option. Instead, evaluate your stand-in foods. Is a frozen yogurt standing in for the ice cream that you really desire? Does the artificial butter in your fridge stand in for real butter? Do you dream of a warm, homemade chocolate chip cookie but settle for the stand-in, fat-free, sugar-free version instead—and sometimes eat the entire box because all the free, low, and faux ingredients leave you feeling unsatisfied?

Review your pantry. Make an honest evaluation and give yourself permission to not pretend to actually like the fake stuff. Be willing to use your God-given brain again, and *get real.*

PRACTICING YOUR FRENCH

This week:

1. Perform a pantry exorcism: Remove all fake foods from your fridge and pantry.
2. Bite into a big juicy apple. Remember the simple pleasure of tasting unadulterated whole food.
3. Shop to restock, purchasing only real food. Eliminate prepared, preserved, or modified choices.

Interlude
Le Pain: Breaking Bread in Paris

WHEN YOU THINK ABOUT France, often bread is the first food to come to mind: specifically, the long, slender loaf called a baguette. What makes the baguette so special is its shape, which allows the maximum amount of dough to be directly exposed to heat during the baking process, producing the thick crust favored by the French. Most baguettes are 2–3 feet long and 3–5 inches thick.

Cornell professor Steven Kaplan, a student of French bread, offers the following description of a well-crafted loaf:

> When you squeeze it, its golden brown crust should crackle and even sing. Its aroma should be a little bit sweet, a little bit toasty. There should be a good marriage between its crust and its interior crumb. When the crumb is pressed, it should spring back rapidly. Its color should be off-white and its cavities widely distributed and uneven in size. Its nutty, buttery taste should be both sweet and savory—like a good chardonnay.*

After the Second World War, standards for French bread declined, mainly due to grain shortages. As a result of these shortages, bread makers lowered their expectations and had to use different baking processes. When bread began to be mass-produced in giant furnaces, standards were compromised even further.

There's good news for lovers of real, old-fashioned French bread—the traditional methods are back! Skilled bakers such as Lionel Poilane, one of France's most famous, have developed methods that ensure quantity and quality.

The French government passed legislation in 1993 designed to prevent any bakery from calling itself a *boulangerie* if it does not make, knead, and cook entirely from scratch on the premises. French food laws define "French" bread as a product containing only flour, water, yeast, and salt. The addition of any other ingredient to the basic recipe requires the baker to use a different name for the final product. There are of course many recipes (using particular flours, varying proportions, a certain type of salt, etc.), but most still adhere to the baguette shape and use a high baking temperature (425 degrees or above).

For the next time you're in Paris, here are some authentic *boulangeries* where you're sure to find a good loaf—a baguette or another of the country's rich variety of traditional breads.

Poilane
8 rue du Cherche-Midi – 75006 Paris
49 blvd. de Grenelle – 75015 Paris
38 rue Debelleyme – 75003 Paris

Lionel Poilane is known throughout the world for his substantial, round, country-style loaf, called a *miche* or a *boule*. No baguettes are baked here, but lots of delectable pastries.

Jean-Luc Poujauran
20 rue Jean-Nicot – 75007 Paris

Celebrated for his excellent country bread, *petits pains aux noix* (walnut rolls), and *fougasse aux olives* (olive bread), Poujauran also offers a few cakes that might include *gateaux basques* and caramel-colored *canneles*.

Rene Saint-Ouen
11 blvd. Haussmann –75008 Paris

The 1997 winner of "The Best Baguette of the Year," Saint-Ouen's crusty loaf was served at the Elysée Palace during Jacque Chirac's presidency.

L'Autre Boulange
43 rue de Montreuil – 75011 Paris

Bio country bread, herb loafs, tomato bread, and other specialty breads are among the offerings at Michel Cousins's establishment.

WHAT TO LOOK FOR IN A BAGUETTE

A good baguette exhibits a perfect balance between the crust,
which must be a rich, dark caramel color, and the soft interior
(*la mie*). A delicate crust, a color similar to fresh hay, and a spotted
underside testify that the bread was cooked in an industrial oven, possibly
from frozen dough. The *mie* of a good baguette is a creamy color and has
large, uneven air holes. The industrial loaf will be
snow-white, with small, even holes. A good baguette's texture
is moist and slightly chewy with a full, almost nutty flavor.

Le Moulin de la Vierge
105 rue Vercingetorix – 75014 Paris
64 rue St Dominique – 75007 Paris
6 rue de Levis – 75017 Paris
166 avenue de Suffren – 75015 Paris

These bakeries owned by Basil Kamir offer excellent breads and
traditional pastries. The olive and anchovy *fougasse*, a provincial-style
flatbread, is exceptionally good.

A la Flûte Gana
226 rue des Pyrenees – 75020 Paris

This shop is named for its trademarked baguette, called *la flûte gana*.
Two daughters now operate the shop their father founded.

Ganachaud
150 rue de Menilmontant – 75020 Paris

Bread connoisseurs particularly favor Ganachaud's delicious country
bread.

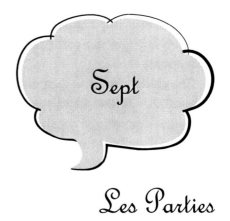

Sept

Les Parties
Portions

Never eat more than you can lift.
—Miss Piggy, Muppet character

THE PARISIAN CAFÉ IS the heartbeat of the city. Agile waiters zoom around small circular tables like human pinballs. The energy of their movement stands in contrast to the deliberate poise of the local diners. And I don't know this for sure, but I doubt that Parisians wear watches.

Here I sit, trying not to stare while still taking in all that this moving picture has to offer. I'm starting to think that, when it comes to weight management, reducing the size of a table makes even more sense than using smaller plates since all of these French men and women are as thin as a pin. The food they order fits perfectly on the surface, with room for an ashtray, a liter of water, and bread and butter—the perfect image of the seventh secret: smaller portions.

While most of the patrons are French, there are a few foreigners. The Americans stand out mainly because they are much louder than the French, plus they order lots more food—so much that it sometimes doesn't fit on the little round tables.

I see a little bit of commotion in my peripheral vision, and again I try not to stare. I'm sure the noise is coming from a table of three overweight Americans. I couldn't help but notice them earlier when I was being seated; they look unusually large on this patio of the fashionably thin, like adults sitting in little kindergarten chairs.

The waiter is doing his best to serve all the food the three had ordered. He had suggested that the meal be enjoyed in courses, but the Americans preferred it served all at once. The waiter, a consummate professional, accommodated the Americans, knowing full well what would happen.

The entire table and a few of the chairs topple over onto the sidewalk, smashing dishes, splashing beverages, and making me wish that at that very moment I could wiggle my American nose and *poof*—I'm French.

A Paradox with a Payback

So what about the cheese, croissants, pastries, butter, cream, and foie gras—not to mention soufflés and duck à l'orange—that would seem, by American standards, to be dietary pitfalls but are cornerstones of the French way of eating? And all the while the French have much less heart disease than Americans. What are the health educators on this side of the Atlantic to say about this paradox?

Clearly, on the surface the French diet would seem to have drawbacks. I mean, they eat nearly four times the butter we Americans consume. The great majority of French people violate the U.S. government's "Diet for a Healthy Heart" guidelines, which call for consuming fewer than 30 percent of calories from fat and fewer than 10 percent of calories from saturated fat.

More specifically, 86 percent of French adults get more than 30 percent of their calories from fat, and a shocking 96 percent obtain more than 10 percent from saturated fat, found in foods like cream cheese, butter, red meat, and foie gras (most French eat about 14–15 percent of calories as saturated fat).

It should come as no revelation, then, that average French blood cholesterol and blood pressure levels are higher than American levels. The average French man's cholesterol is 218–252 (depending on the area of France he is from), compared with 209 in the United States. French women's cholesterol levels are about the same as those of French men. But the French have a much lower rate of death due to heart disease than Americans. They are two and a half times less likely to die of heart disease than we are.

"Just on the basis of higher cholesterol levels and blood pressure readings, the death rate from heart disease in France should be much higher," says Michael H.

Criqui, MD, professor of family and preventative medicine at the University of California, San Diego.* Fascinated by the French Paradox because of his interest in how alcohol affects health, Dr. Criqui concluded that moderate wine consumption plays at least some role in explaining this health marvel, but there is so much more in the way of explaining the excellent health of the French.

At this halfway point in the book and before we consider more specifically the portion distortion that is a major culprit in the fattening of Americans, let's review some of the nutritional principles at the heart of the French way of eating—principles that can put you in line for the benefits it confers.

The Pleasure of Your Company

Almost nowhere in France will you see people eating on the go. Most often the French sit down for no less than an hour and enjoy their meal and the company—even if that's just a magazine article or their own thoughts. I firmly believe that one of the reasons the French have a lower rate of death from heart attack is the stress-relieving advantage of an extended, pleasurable, and fulfilling mealtime.

Remember, at some point in the future when the headlines report that science validates the relaxation factor at mealtime as a significant component to a healthy heart, a healthy overall diet, and a healthy metabolism—you read it here first!

Mediterranean Links

Cheese, pastry, and croissants aside, the French eat pretty much a Mediterranean diet. And while they consume more red meat than, say, the Italians or Greeks, the meat is more of a garnish (think vegetable stew with beef rather than beef stew with vegetables) rather than the focus of the meal, as is traditional in the United States.

I'll let you in on a big secret that helps explain the French Paradox and, while we're at it, the benefits of the Mediterranean diet, too. The French eat mountains more fruits and vegetables than we Americans do. "Shopping for fresh produce is an important part of almost every day," says chef Alain Sailhac, provost and senior dean of Culinary Studies at the French Culinary Institute. "People choose fresh produce every day and then build a meal around those items. . . . As a result of their focus on fruits and vegetables, the French typically eat more than five servings of fruits and vegetables daily. In contrast, Americans eat just three."*

Like their Mediterranean friends, the French enjoy liberal helpings of olive oil. They eat several fish dishes a week and plenty of whole grains and beans. Herbs are a key element of French cooking, and then, of course, there's the famous glass of wine at each meal.

Is It the Wine or the Flavonoids in the Wine?

"Several aspects of the French diet could explain the French paradox," says Edwin Frankel, adjunct professor of food science and technology at the University of California at Davis. "When we first heard about the French paradox, my colleagues and I wondered if flavonoids, the phytochemicals that are particularly high in red wine, could be at least partly responsible for the protection against heart disease. It makes sense that something besides alcohol accounts for the beneficial effect of red wine," he says. "Research suggests that something besides alcohol in wine, especially red wine, is significantly superior to alcohol provided by other beverages, such as beer or whiskey. It seems that phenolic antioxidants may be conferring this benefit."* (Phenolics, including flavonoids, are a type of phytochemical.)

Researchers from around the world learned that red wine solids stripped of their alcohol content (in other words, natural 100 percent grape juice) were able to stop platelet clumping. From the laboratory of flavonoids researcher John Folts, professor of medicine and head of the coronary thrombosis research lab at the University of Wisconsin School of Medicine in Madison, more evidence proved that the heart-protective property of red wine had little to do with alcohol.

Dr. Folts was able to discern that pure alcohol stopped platelet clumping, but only when blood alcohol reached 0.2 (that's double the legal limit for intoxication of 0.1). Red wine came through when blood alcohol was a mere 0.03—in all probability because it contains flavonoids.*

Phytochemicals in fruits and vegetables help ward off heart disease because they are very potent antioxidants. As with all living things, we humans require oxygen to exist, but the process of using oxygen creates oxygen by-products called free radicals—unstable particles that move from cell to cell in an effort to stabilize themselves and in the process leave a path of damage.

When it comes to the heart, free radicals are responsible for several damaging actions. First, they change the body's protective HDL levels through oxidation, and oxidized LDL (the "bad" cholesterol) swells and lodges in the arteries. Free radicals also alter platelet function, making it more likely that platelets will clump together and clog arteries.

"Although the body has its own system of scavenging free radicals, it needs help from the outside," says Edwin Frankel. "There is considerable evidence that flavonoids and other phytochemicals in fruits and vegetables are powerful antioxidants."* These plant-based antioxidants can stop platelets from clumping and LDL from oxidizing and clogging artery walls. And flavonoids reduce

AN AMERICAN IN PARIS: DAILY LIFE

Susan felt very safe and relaxed in Paris. "My husband and I would walk home at two in the morning and never feel threatened in any way. Or I would take the metro home late at night and then walk the few blocks to my apartment, never once feeling afraid to be walking alone."

She talked about her sense of adventure and freedom while she lived in Paris. "I felt very alive in France," she shared. "Every day I found a different route to the market, or to a friend's home or to nowhere in particular, and I would always discover an enchanting fountain, garden, or architectural detail on a building that I had never noticed before. Paris is a visual feast!"

Susan was devoted to her work as a freelance producer. I knew this firsthand, having had the pleasure of working with her on a few productions, and, like most Americans, her professional position defined a good part of her life.

"This was the first time I had not worked in years, and I was afraid that I would miss that pace and sense of purpose," she revealed. "But that fear quickly dissipated. I just loved not having the stress of it all. I was never bored, and Paris offered me the opportunity to discover myself all over again in a new way."

"After spending a few years in France, what do you think the French do better than Americans?" I asked.

Without even a slight pause, Susan replied, "The French know how to slow down and enjoy life and family. They realize it's okay to just sit and read a book along the Seine, take a stroll around the park, or relax and enjoy their food and the company of family and friends."

Like Carolyn (from chapter 3), Susan noted that this was most apparent on Sundays. "It was always quiet until later in the afternoon. Then everyone seemed to come out in force, children and parents playing in the park, walking along the streets, stopping to talk to neighbors. Sunday was truly the day of rest," she recalled fondly.

inflammation and thus the narrowing of blood vessels, another culprit in the clogging of arteries.

Where do we get flavonoids? (Take note: Wine is *not* at the top of the list.)

- ⋙ The absolute best sources: onions, kale, green beans, broccoli, endive, celery, cranberries, and citrus fruits.
- ⋙ Moderately good sources: red wine, tea, lettuce, tomatoes, red peppers, fava beans, strawberries, apples, grape juice, and tomato juice.
- ⋙ Low-level sources: cabbage, carrots, mushrooms, peas, spinach, peaches, white wine, coffee, and orange juice.

It All Relates to What's on Your Plate

The produce you choose every day as you plan your meals is chock-full of a variety of other beneficial phytochemicals besides flavonoids. Sweet potatoes, red bell peppers, spinach, kale, cantaloupe, peaches, and apricots are known for their high levels of carotenoid, a phytochemical known to reduce cholesterol.

Garlic, onions, and shallots, members of the allium family, offer another group of phytochemicals called organosulfur compounds that help stop platelet clumping by reducing platelet stickiness.

Other phytochemicals—the tocotrienols, abundant in grains—seem to limit the oxidation of LDL cholesterol, in addition to helping reduce the body's creation of cholesterol. Lentils, dried beans, and peas (staples of the French and Mediterranean diets) contain the phytochemicals called saponins, known to bind cholesterol from the intestinal tract and escort it out of the body unabsorbed.

Olive oil contains at least two phytochemicals that have been identified as protective against heart disease. Just as with the flavonoids in red wine, olive oil phytochemicals contain phenolic compounds; they work in the same way to protect LDLs from oxidation. Stick with extra-virgin olive oil, as the French do, since it has the most phenolic compounds.

Fish, which the French typically eat several times a week, may lower the risk of heart attack in at least three ways. Fish contain polyunsaturated fatty acids called omega-3s that prevent platelet clumping, keep HDL cholesterol levels healthfully high, especially in women, and help the heart beat in a steady, healthy rhythm.

Dietary Diversity

Eat a varied diet by following this simple rule: Make sure your plate contains lots of different colors. A colorful array of foods not only ensures that you are getting plenty of phytochemicals but also that you are getting a wide variety of them—what nutritionists call dietary diversity.

Diversity is important because yellow tomatoes, for example, have different phytochemicals than those found in orange and red ones, as do the different types of salad greens. The French shop more often than we do here, buying smaller quantities of the freshest produce they can find, and they tend to have a more adventuresome palate, while we Americans tend to buy the same food items over and over again. Eating many different kinds of foods is not only fun, it helps you take in more of the beneficial chemicals and nutrients that foods deliver.

Portion Distortion

> *In eating, a third of the stomach should be filled with food, a third with drink, and the rest left empty.*
> —The Talmud

To some extent, the French Paradox can be explained by the fact that French portions are notably smaller than American portions. Yes, the French diet is rich in butter, cream, pastry, and cheese, but studies have shown that the French consume fewer calories than Americans do, and the result is a smaller number of overweight and obese people.

For example, the standard individual portion of yogurt sold in France is 4.5 ounces, while the standard size in America is 7.94 ounces.

A joint French-American team of scientists from France's Centre National de la Recherche Scientifique (National Center of Scientific Research) and the University of Pennsylvania set out in 2003 to test the hypothesis that the French eat less and consume smaller portions than Americans. Researchers weighed portions at eleven similar restaurants in Paris and Philadelphia and found that:

- ❧ The average entrée portion size in Paris was 25 percent smaller than in Philadelphia (9.78 ounces versus 12.21 ounces).
- ❧ Chinese restaurants in Philadelphia served dishes that were 72 percent larger than in Parisian Chinese food restaurants.

- A candy bar in Philadelphia was 41 percent larger than the same candy bar in Paris.
- A soft drink was 53 percent larger and a hot dog was 63 percent larger in Philadelphia than in France.

I wrote earlier in the book about how real food gets to the heart of our hunger, whereas fake, fat-free concoctions leave us growling for more. This may explain the "just one more" fat-free, sugar-free cookie syndrome compared to the "ummm . . . that was yummy" satisfaction of one delicious, homemade confection.

SERVINGS SHORTCUTS

Don't worry about measuring servings precisely.
Here are three easy ways to think about serving sizes:

1/2 cup (4 fluid ounces)	a closed fist
1 cup (8 fluid ounces)	a softball
3 ounces (of fish or meat)	a deck of cards

How much is enough? It seems like common sense that one whole apple or banana equals a portion, but this misconception about serving size can sabotage your weight-management efforts. Become portion proficient and know when enough is enough.

1 cup leafy vegetables
1 large carrot
1/2 cup cooked or chopped raw or canned fruit or vegetables
1/2 large apple, banana, or orange, or grapefruit
3/4 cup vegetable or fruit juice
1/2 cup cooked cereal or pasta
1 ounce ready-to-eat cereal
1 slice of bread or half a bagel
1 1/2 ounces cheese

1 cup milk
1 cup yogurt
1/2 cup cooked beans
3 ounces tofu
3 ounces cooked fish
2–3 ounces organic, cooked poultry
2–3 ounces lean, organic meat
1 whole organic egg
1 teaspoon canola, olive, or flaxseed oil
2 tablespoons chopped nuts or nut butter

Keep it simple, healthy, and French by eating modest serving sizes, like the ones shown above, and by using the three-quarters rule: Fill your plate with three-quarters plant foods and one-quarter animal food, plus a serving of healthy oil, avocado, or nuts. Enjoy a glass of wine and top the meal off with an ounce of fine chocolate, and you're well on your way to optimum health and a smaller waistline.

Size Does Matter

Yvette and Aubert had arrived at their new home in the United States from Georgia, a country in the Caucasus region at the eastern end of the Black Sea, with Turkey and Armenia to the south, Azerbaijan to the east, and Russia to the north, across the Caucasus Mountains.

Georgia is considered the breadbasket of its region because of the richness of its soil and an advantageous climate. It's said that the fruit and vegetables the Georgians grow, which practically burst at the seams with flavor, will spoil your taste buds forever. The fable of God tripping on the Caucasus Mountains and dropping his lunch there is one explanation, but most give credit to the richness of the soil and the absence of processed foods.

A meal of tomatoes, fresh cheese, *puri* (bread), and fruit is one of the best repasts to enjoy in this region. And it's very inexpensive; you can buy fruits and vegetables in the market for a mere fraction of what you would pay in the United States. Georgian cuisine is prepared from scratch with fresh, locally grown products; supermarkets have barely touched this country.

"When we first arrived we were able to finish only a slice of pizza," Yvette explained.

"Now we eat the whole pizza," Aubert added.

After just a few months in the United States, Yvette and Aubert each had gained twenty-five pounds. They had come to my office to design my business website, but before we realized it we were in a nutritional session. They committed to working as a couple to shed the pounds together in a reasonable manner. The more I coached them, the more homesick they felt, until one day Yvette declared, "This is exactly how we ate in our country. I don't know what happened to us here. We know all of this, and somehow we've gotten completely off track."

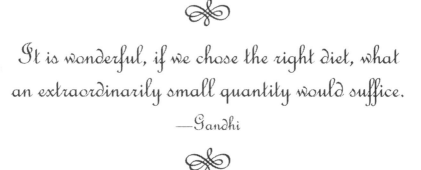

It is wonderful, if we chose the right diet, what an extraordinarily small quantity would suffice.

—Gandhi

I reflected on my days hosting foreign exchange students and remembered the weight that most of the kids gained while here in the States. Fast food was new, abundant, and seductive for them; in their home countries most didn't have access to pizza, McDonald's, or Taco Bell. If they did, the portions in the U.S. were supersized, plus there was a fast-food option on every corner. Over the course of a year they typically gained new (and bad) habits, along with ten pounds.

The same thing was happening to Yvette and Aubert. In Georgia they ate locally grown, whole foods, and their neighbors shared their values. Eating was not a national pastime. Portions were small, healthy, and realistic. In the United States the couple's new friends and neighbors exhibit a different attitude toward food and eating. Much of the food is unwholesome and fake, portions are gigantic, and when there's nothing better to do, people eat.

Yvette and Aubert fell victim to their new environment. Before they knew it, their eyes had adjusted to larger serving sizes, their stomachs were accommodating larger portions, and their taste for junk food was turned on.

Still, they had an edge over most people; they could recognize the difference between high- and low-quality food, could spot fake food, and knew from their own experience that they could be satisfied and well nourished by smaller portions. And they knew how much better they felt (and looked) when they adhered to their native customs.

After a few sessions in my office and a trip or two to Whole Foods, they got back on track. In a very short time they lost twenty-five pounds each—without dieting. Of course, Aubert lost it quickly, reinforcing the research that on average the metabolism of a man is 5 to 10 percent higher than that of a woman of the same weight and height, attributed in part to men having more lean muscle mass.* Who said life is fair? This could have irritated Yvette, but instead it motivated her, and very soon they were both back to their natural weight.

Yvette and Aubert had a point of reference—the positive eating patterns established in their childhoods were easy and comfortable to fall back into. For those of us born and raised in the United States, adapting our eating habits to be more like those of people who grew up in Europe, where portion control is handed down like a birthright, may seem difficult and awkward initially.

Here are some ideas to set you off in the right direction. To help your eyes get a general picture of the size of your stomach, open your fist so that the tips of the thumb and forefinger touch. Your stomach is about the width of this open fist and twice as long. Notice how small individuals have smaller fists and larger individuals larger fists. We know from the discussion of the basal metabolic rate in the first chapter that an individual of large stature requires more calories than one of small stature.

The next time you approach a meal, check the fist against the dish. Create a visual image of the food entering your stomach, remaining constantly aware of the size of the vessel you are filling (and hopefully not expanding). At the same time, remember that in order to digest your food effectively (that means no heartburn or bloated feeling), you must eat slowly, chew your food, and eat until you are about 80 percent sated—a point at which you will be satisfied, but not stuffed. This may take some getting used to, but hang in there.

If you are following these guidelines, chances are you'll be eating about half the food you are accustomed to. But you'll be replacing quantity with quality—tasty, satisfying food.

Once you have established this new, healthy pattern, you will notice subtle differences in your hunger at different points throughout the day. Adjust accordingly. Let's say you've enjoyed a wonderful lunch out with a friend; that evening, it may be that a lighter dinner of soup and salad is best. I make adjustments like this on any given day, depending on my activity level. In no time at all you'll become aware of the needs of your body and will find yourself naturally ebbing and flowing along with your metabolism.

Here Today, More Tomorrow

Every dieter knows that practical steps are a very small part of a successful weight management outcome. The 800-pound gorilla in the room is the sense of deprivation. Most diets fail because a deprivation mind-set is contradictory to the way most people want to live.

We are not robots. We are human beings with *appetites* for a variety of tastes and life experiences.

One crippling response to deprivation is fear that our favorite food choices are no longer and will no longer be available to us. (Remember Blanche and "I can never eat carbs again"?) That fear is at the heart of countless failed diets, destructive bouts of binge eating, the roller coaster of weight gain, weight loss, weight gain, weight loss.

Instead, why not abolish the diet and accept that the foods humans have eaten for generations are here to stay, and that the food that is here today *will* be here tomorrow and the next day and the next day? Such acceptance creates an inner climate of peace, freedom, and stability that supports optimum health and weight management. Eat the foods that you like—in balance and moderation—and repeat tomorrow. Unless you are on death row, there is no one last meal.

PRACTICING YOUR FRENCH

This week:

1. The next time you eat in a restaurant, eat half of what you are served and wait a few minutes. Are you satisfied with half? If so, box up the rest for another meal.
2. In a restaurant, order appetizer portions. Again, ask yourself if this smaller portion satisfies your hunger. If not, consider sharing dessert with your dining partner or order a cappuccino to finish off the meal.
3. Be less possessive with your food. Use any cooking or dining occasion as an opportunity to share something from your plate or kitchen.

Interlude
Le Chocolat and
How the French Came to Love It

MEXICAN MYTHOLOGY tells us that our age-old obsession with chocolate is one we share with the gods who consumed chocolate in Paradise. The seed of the chocolate tree was bestowed upon man as a special blessing by the God of the Air. All this is quite believable indeed if you've ever savored a divine piece of really good chocolate.

It seems that every culture wants some credit for their influence on chocolate. In most accounts chocolate appeared on the scene around 600 A.D., when the Mayans migrated into the northern regions of South America and developed some of the earliest known cocoa-tree (or cacao-tree) plantations in the Yucatan Peninsula.

Ancient chronicles show that the Aztecs believed in a god that traveled to earth on a beam of the morning star with a cocoa tree from Paradise and offered it to the inhabitants. The natives learned how to roast and grind the precious seeds, making a paste that dissolved in water. They added spices and called this drink *chocolatl*, meaning "bitter water." They credited the bitter water with bringing universal wisdom and knowledge. Well, there you go—another good reason to eat chocolate!

The ancient Mexicans believed that the goddesses of food and water were also the guardian goddesses of cocoa. Every year a human sacrifice was performed for the goddesses, and the victim's last meal always included cocoa.

In 1519 Spanish explorer Hernando Cortez visited the court of the Mexican emperor Montezuma and drank *chocolatl*, flavored with spices and served in goblets as an aphrodisiac. In 1528 Cortez took chocolate back to Spain, hiding it away in Spanish monasteries for nearly a century. The monks eventually created a profitable chocolate industry for Spain, which monopolized the trade by planting cocoa trees in its overseas colonies.

It was an Italian traveler, Antonio Carletti, who in 1606 discovered the secret of this chocolate treasure and introduced cocoa to other parts of Europe. Thus the Spanish monopoly on the chocolate trade ended. Within just a few years the news of chocolate had spread across Italy, Germany, England—and France. In the early 1600s Jewish immigrants, driven out of Spain, brought chocolate to the port city of Bayonne in southwestern France.

Princess Maria Theresa's betrothal to Louis XIV in 1615 offered the French court an ideal opportunity to fully embrace chocolate. The Spanish princess's engagement gift to her fiancé was most precious to her—cocoa beans packaged in an elegantly ornate chest. Along with the beans came her chocolate-loving ladies-in-waiting and a crew of retainers charged with making her favorite indulgence—hot chocolate. This royal marriage was made in heaven, with chocolate as a reigning symbol of the combined cultures of France and Spain.

YOU SAY COCOA, I SAY CACAO

The official name of the chocolate tree is *Theobroma cacao*. Over the years, people have replaced "cacao" (pronounced ka-kow) with the Anglicized word "cocoa." Most of us grew up saying "cocoa bean," not "cacao bean." Now, with the rebirth of old-style, artisanal chocolate, there is a movement to reclaim the bean's rightful name: cacao.

Hot chocolate was extremely popular with Louis XIV, who reigned as the Sun King for seventy-two years (1643–1715), and the members of his court at Versailles. The king's personal recipe included an egg yolk to guarantee a rich, thick concoction. He appointed Sieur David Illou to manufacture and sell chocolate, which not only created a new commercial product for the French economy but also allegedly inspired erotic pleasures. It was said that in Louis's seventy-second year he was making love to his wife twice a day . . . perhaps the effect of chocolate?

Chocolate's reputation as an aphrodisiac flourished in the French courts. In the visual arts and literature erotic imagery inspired by chocolate was common. Casanova was reputed to use chocolate, along with champagne, as part of his many conquests. Later the Marquis de Sade became proficient in using chocolate to disguise poisons. Madame de Pompadour was advised to use chocolate with ambergris to stimulate her desire for Louis XV . . . but to no avail. Madame du Barry, reputed to be nymphomaniacal, encouraged her lovers to drink chocolate in order to keep up with her.

In 1657 even the British succumbed when a Frenchman opened London's first chocolate shop. Such venues became trendy spots where members of elite London society met to drink and savor the new luxury food.

Just to be sure that every culture gets proper credit, let me mention that in the 1700s Swedish naturalist Carolus Linnaeus, who designed the modern naming system for plants and animals, expanded the name to *Theobroma cacao*; the first word is Greek for "food of the gods."

In 1844 a Dutch man, J. S. Fry, and his sons were the first to make hardened eating cocoa. And as they say, the rest is history. ❦

Huit

Le Métabolisme
Metabolism

Do you know how to digest your food? Do you know how to fill your lungs with air? Do you know how to establish, regulate, and direct the metabolism of your body—the assimilation of foodstuff so that it builds muscles, bones, and flesh? No, you don't know how consciously, but there is a wisdom within you that does know.

—Donald Curtis, inspirational speaker and writer

THE EIGHTH SECRET: Metabolism is the sum total of *all* the chemical reactions in the body. Most of us think of metabolism only as a calorie-burning phenomenon—a body process that relates to thermic efficiency. But this definition alone is inadequate. Relying on it may explain why the approaches to metabolism we are accustomed to, such as exercise and supplements that "kick-start" it, are not effective.

Metabolism does not occur in the body alone. It operates equally and simultaneously in body, mind, emotions, and spirit. If something is truly nourishing for the soul, then it is quite factually nourishing for the body. That nourishment is what fuels metabolism.

Eating to the Beat of Our Digestive Rhythms

By measuring temperature in the human body we are able to also measure metabolism. The "hotter" we are the more metabolic we are.

Body temperature has a rhythm that is predictable and very much in sync with the cosmos. During the overnight and early-morning hours, while we sleep our body temperature drops. In our sleep state we are in a state of rest, healing, and repair. We burn calories while we are sleeping, just not as many as we do when we're awake.

Assuming you don't consume a large meal before going to sleep, you are in a fasting state overnight. The minute your eyes pop open in the morning, your body temperature begins to rise. You wake up right along with your metabolism. Even if you stayed in bed all day and didn't move, your temperature and metabolism would still rise because our bodies are programmed to mirror the rhythms of the sun in its apparent daily journey across the sky.

Because the body's heat naturally rises in the morning, eating at this time is a good idea—you will be providing your body with the nutrients it is ready to process. Adding fuel, in the form of food, to your body's furnace will cause its temperature to remain high and even rise higher. The body's temperature continues to rise slowly and steadily until it peaks around noon, reaching its apex as the sun attains its highest point in the sky. Our digestive force is the hottest at lunchtime—a scientific fact that reinforces the fact that we have a profound connection to the universe.

That's why it's smart to enjoy our largest meal during this window of time. Once again, science validates the French and their custom of taking a break between the hours of 12 noon and 2:00 P.M., when they eat the largest meal of the day. They are honoring and working with the natural rhythms of the body.

Between roughly 4:00 P.M. and 6:00 P.M. the body's temperature starts to rise again—just in time for *le goûter*. It's no coincidence that, after indulging in a small snack, we begin to feel our energy return and experience a "second wind" after an early-afternoon slump.

AN AMERICAN IN PARIS:
A CULTURE CENTERED AROUND FOOD

"Food is such a big part of the French culture. We were often invited to the home of our French friends, Jean-Pierre and Kathleen, for Sunday lunch. It would start around 1 p.m. and last until 5 p.m., always beginning with champagne and nuts and olives," Susan told me. "Next came a lovely meat dish prepared by Jean-Pierre, a hunter as well as a cook; one never knew what he would prepare. The meal always included fresh vegetables and bread, often soup, and then salad *après*. Then cheese and more bread, and more wine and then dessert and then coffee and then a digestive.

"Conversations would run the gamut. The French are not embarrassed to discuss anything. It was always interesting and fun, and the intercultural atmosphere was stimulating," Susan reminisced.

"It was great walking home afterward," Susan remembered, "and the nice long stroll would make us feel we were working off all that rich food. But the reality is, we never felt overly full—an odd phenomenon when you consider how much we consumed. But it did take us a full four hours, if not longer, to complete the meal.

"I loved dining in Paris, especially at our French friends' homes. I learned how easy it is to entertain, and I do so more now since I have returned," she added.

Most of the French have dined by 8:00 p.m., in time for another downward trend in temperature at around 9:00 p.m., in preparation for falling asleep. Sleep research proves that we cannot fall asleep soundly unless our body temperature is dropping. Because eating raises the body's temperature, a big meal before bed interferes with a restful sleep.

Sleep: A Time for Cleansing and Repair

I love to sleep—I really *love* it! I try very hard not to consume a large volume of food before sleep because I don't want to miss the great metabolic gifts of slumber.

During the night the body shifts most of its metabolic energy to maintenance, detoxification, repair, and growth of its tissues and organs. When you grow new muscle and bone, you do so during sleep. The liver, the largest organ in the body and a cleansing organ, does most of its work in the late-evening and early-morning hours.

Here's a fact that's essential for you to know about the way the body operates: Short-term survival needs take precedence over long-term needs. So if you eat a large meal before bedtime, the energy needed for detoxification, repair, and maintenance is re-routed to digestion, and you lose all of the important benefits of sleep. That's why when you eat a large meal late in the evening, you feel congested and heavy when you wake up in the morning—you didn't detoxify during the night.

The period between dinner and breakfast is a fast, engineered into our bodies by eons of evolution and designed to allow a period for rebuilding the body. Waking up in a toxic state, skipping breakfast, eating on the run during the day, and then repeating the cycle creates an arrhythmic pattern—and denies your body the renovation it requires.

Cutting back on sleep reduces the benefits of dieting, according to a study published in October 2010 in the *Annals of Internal Medicine*.* One of the study's authors, Plamen Penev, assistant professor of medicine at the University of Chicago, said, "If your goal is to lose fat, skipping sleep is like poking sticks in your bicycle wheels. Cutting back on sleep, a behavior that is ubiquitous in modern society, appears to compromise efforts to lose fat through dieting. In our study it reduced fat loss by 55 percent."

On the *Today* show on October 20, 2010, Ann Curry interviewed Keri Glassman, a registered dietician and a contributing editor of *Women's Health* magazine, who reported that getting fewer than seven hours of sleep increases appetite and the risk of obesity. More specifically, six hours of sleep increases obesity by 23 percent, and five hours of sleep increases obesity by 50 percent.

Here's why. Getting less than seven hours of sleep increases the hunger hormone ghrelin and decreases the fullness hormone leptin. Leptin levels tell the brain when the body does or doesn't need more food. The hormone ghrelin makes one hungry, slows metabolism, and decreases the body's ability to burn fat. Want to stop feeling hungry? Nighty-night!

Hunger Is Healthy

If you're in an arrhythmic cycle, it's easy enough to retrain your body and to restore a healthy lifestyle and metabolism. Until recently I lived in a very hot climate; temperatures often reached the high 80s by the time I was ready for my morning walk, so I tended to eat a light breakfast of cereal, milk, and berries. I am generally hungry in the morning since I don't eat a large meal in the evening, and I really look forward to my breakfast.

Remember, hunger is, simply stated, a signal from your body's intelligence center that it wants to eat and is prepared for the proper metabolism of food. Hunger is healthy; ignoring it is not commendable and may create a *hypo-metabolic* mode (in other words, a lower or slower metabolism). In this mode, brought on by the body's fear of starvation, our metabolism stores the majority of incoming calories as fat instead of burning them for energy.

I tend to be an early riser and enjoy a three-mile walk with my dogs each and every morning. Afterward, I can feel that my hunger and metabolism are both on the rise. You too will notice this once you become aware of your body's cycle and respect its natural rhythms. As I begin to look forward to my main meal, I consider my options. Know how you think about a favorite food and your mouth starts watering? That's the method I use to determine what my meal will be.

Sometimes my mouth isn't exactly watering at the same time my stomach is growling. That's when I take a minute, slow down, and ask myself, "Do I have a craving for something crunchy, cold, and refreshing or maybe something warm, smooth, and comforting? Do simple flavors speak to me, or am I more in the mood for something spicy and complex?"

Finally, the dish that sounds the best—that seems it would most please my taste buds, that makes my mouth water, literally or figuratively—is the one I choose. This technique has proved to be a great way for me to cut through any diet-mentality mental gymnastics and uncover my true food yearnings.

Awareness Helps Regulate Metabolism

The scientific term for "mouth watering" is *cephalic phase digestive response* (CPDR; *cephalic* means "relating to the head"). Digestion begins in the head as chemical and mechanical receptors on the tongue and the mouth and nasal cavities are stimulated by thinking about food and then seeing food, smelling it, tasting it, and chewing it.

The process of what I like to call "staying awake at the plate"—paying attention to those receptors and the messages they are sending—initiates the secretion of saliva, gastric acid and enzymes, and gut-associated neuropeptides, as well as the production of a full range of pancreatic enzymes, including trypsin, chymotrypsin, pancreatic amylase, and lipase—all working together, assisting in breaking your food down so that your cells get the nutrients they need.

Staying awake at the plate also causes blood to rush to the digestive organs, the stomach and intestines to rhythmically contract, and electrolyte concentrations throughout the digestive tract to shift in preparation for incoming food.

Scientists say that 30 to 40 percent of our total digestive response to any meal is due to the CPDR. If we are asleep at the plate and fail to register our hunger, visual interest, or a sense of taste, smell, and satisfaction, then we are metabolizing our meal at only 60 to 70 percent efficiency. Lack of attention means decreased blood flow to the digestive organs, less oxygenation, and finally, a weakened metabolic force—exactly what we don't want.

The French, by way of their culinary traditions and respect for food, naturally dine with awareness. Most have been raised in an environment in which a car or the area in front of a television set are not considered proper dining venues. Their CPDR is in order.

When the French finish a meal, they are completely satiated because they have been completely present. In contrast, eating while watching television, for example, or in some other way not paying attention to what you are eating can leave your belly full but your mouth still hungry.

The important thing to know is that the CPDR is not merely a response but a full-blown requirement. Your brain must experience taste, pleasure, aroma, and satisfaction so it can accurately assess a meal and catalyze your most efficient digestive forces. You may think you have an overeating problem when in fact you are simply not aware of your meal. You are genetically designed to be fulfilled, which involves honoring your body and your appetite with the respect it deserves.

It wasn't until I stopped fantasizing about cake and ice cream and *ate the cake and ice cream* in complete awareness and delight that I was able to move on. I know that this is a radical concept for many of you. We have been conditioned to believe that to lose weight we must deny ourselves food and pleasure, that we must wage war against our appetites. However, fighting the biology of our bodies has not worked for most of us.

If there is a French Paradox, awareness should get much more credit than red wine. Part of that awareness is welcoming hunger, indulging it sensibly, and, in doing so, helping make your metabolism healthy.

BIG NEWS

On June 29, 2010, the news service HealthDay cited a report that obesity rates in 28 states had jumped: "More than two-thirds of states now have adult obesity rates above 25 percent."* "Back in 1991 . . . not a single state had an obesity rate above 20 percent," according to Jeff Levi, executive director of the Trust for America's Health, which co-authored the report with the Robert Wood Johnson Foundation.

Mississippi was the fattest state (33.8 percent of adults are obese), while Alabama and Tennessee tied for second (31.6 percent). The others in the top ten were West Virginia, Louisiana, Oklahoma, Kentucky, Arkansas, South Carolina, and Michigan, tying with North Carolina for 10th place (29.4 percent). The healthiest states in terms of weight were in the Northeast and West. But even in Colorado, the slimmest state, 19.1 percent of people were obese.

More than 35 percent of adults who make less than $15,000 a year were obese versus 24.5 percent who make more than $50,000. Blacks and Latinos outweighed whites in at least 40 states plus D.C., making them more likely to develop diabetes, high blood pressure, and other risk factors for heart disease.

"The link between poverty, race, and obesity is undeniable," Angela Glover Blackwell, founder of the action institute PolicyLink, said in commenting on the report. "For example, Mississippi, the poorest state in nation with an African-American population of more than 37 percent, has the highest obesity rate of any state and highest proportion of obese children." Poor and minority neighborhoods lack safe areas in which to exercise, and many are also "food deserts."

The report also noted that 16.4 percent of children aged 10 to 17 are obese and 18.2 percent are overweight. But we do seem to be paying attention where our children are concerned: 80 percent of Americans say they believe "childhood obesity is a significant and growing challenge for the country."

Metabolism and Exercise

I met Joséphine at a kickboxing class years ago. She worked out every day of the week, one day kickboxing, another with a personal trainer, sweating and sculpting the next day, and so on. In addition, Joséphine employed a personal chef for her family and ate only calorie-controlled, healthy meals.

Yet she looked nothing like an athlete who focused on health in planning her meals. Short in stature, Joséphine was somewhat overweight—and very frustrated. She came to my office for a consultation.

I had a suspicion after seeing the intensity of her exercise program that she was quite possibly wearing herself down and that her metabolism had become locked into a survival mode in which she stored fat instead of muscle. I mentioned this concept to her, which didn't go over very well since she was most definitely committed to the "calories in versus calories out equals body weight" formula.

"But then how is it, Joséphine, that based on your math you haven't lost any weight?" I asked.

"I don't know," she answered. "That's why I'm here." I told her about the findings of Kenneth Cooper, MD. Once a proponent of intense workouts, he eventually did a total about-face concerning vigorous aerobic exercise. His findings at the Cooper Aerobics Center, in Dallas, Texas, showed that low- to moderate-intensity exercise for only thirty minutes three to four times a week was the best prescription for maintaining health, weight, and fitness.

Once I had Joséphine's attention, I questioned her about why she worked out as strenuously as she did. She told me that she hated being short and had never embraced her stature, and that she detested exercise almost as much. I came to the conclusion that she experienced exercise as punishment of her body, which retaliated with a stress response.

Because what Joséphine was doing clearly didn't suit her body type—her weight was proof enough—she agreed to cut back on her exercising from six days to three days a week. Without changing any other habit, she lost nine pounds in two months.

Exercise is not bad, but healthy habits driven by fear, anger, or resentment are not healthy and will not produce results.

Self-limiting thoughts suppress metabolism. I know, based on my own experience. While training for a half-marathon, I was required to record a qualifying 5K time in order to determine what my group training assignment would be. Unfortunately, I didn't think the whole situation through, so I ran like a madwoman and clocked a time well above my normal running speed. I was as proud as a peacock, albeit briefly.

When I showed up the next week to meet my group, I found myself the only woman on the team other than the group's leader, a female elite athlete. I ran with an ex-marine, a twenty-something Rambo type, an iron man, and a frequent marathoner. All my gal pals were in other groups. Seriously, I almost killed myself running that summer.

On Saturday mornings we ran at 5:30 A.M. (usually 5 to 7 miles), in addition to daily track outings, and every so often we were challenged by a longer weekend run of up to 13 miles. Even on the lower-mileage and track days I returned home for a nap, groaning all the way as my sore hipbones ached and throbbed with pain.

On one of the 13-mile hill-training excursions, the ex-marine and I got off course from the group and ended up running 2 additional miles. The following day, as I dashed through the airport in my high heels, I felt my Achilles tendon snap; the pain was riveting. So much for the marathon. But the whole time I had trained I had thought it odd that I had dropped nary a pound.

I'm really not sure what I was trying to prove, but mentally things were off. I was certainly not enjoying the process. I missed my buddies, and the group I had gotten myself into because of my distorted ego and superwoman effort was certainly not at all in tandem with my natural ability.

Secretly, despite the pain, I was happy that the injury gave me an excuse to bag the race. In the weeks that followed I limped around, unable to participate in any aerobic exercise, and I lost seven pounds.

For those of you who doubt the mind–body connection, specifically the mind–metabolism connection, take note. In 1983 medical researchers were testing a new chemotherapy treatment.* One group of cancer patients received the drug being tested, while the other group received a neutral chemical substance—a placebo. Thirty-one percent of the patients on the placebo lost their hair for one reason and one reason only—their own mind and the power of expectation. Because they associated chemotherapy with hair loss, they did, in fact, lose their hair.

Think about it: If the power of thought can result in hair loss, what do you think happens when you eat a delicious ice cream cone, all the while fearing and imagining that you're packing on the pounds? Or what's the result when, like Joséphine, you exercise based on hatred of your body and unknowingly initiate a survival metabolism rather than a metabolically charged pleasure center?

The placebo effect is commonplace; you've heard about it but probably never made the connection between placebo power and food. Simply stated, the placebo effect is your metabolism responding to thoughts, feelings, and expectations. Everything that we *believe* is translated into the body through nerve pathways, the endocrine system, the circulation of neuropeptides (hormones secreted by nervous tissue), the immune network, and the digestive tract.

In our culture we are conditioned to worry about carbohydrates, fat, and sugar. Missing just one day of vigorous aerobic activity throws us into a guilt trip that would make any mother proud. We often forget that we are the masters of our minds and our metabolisms.

PRACTICING YOUR FRENCH

This week:

1. Many people who are accustomed to dieting ignore their body's signals and find it difficult to recognize that they are hungry. Likewise, those who eat past the point when they are hungry may not have discerned true hunger for many years. Make the effort to tune in and become aware of the times when you neglect sensations in your stomach or find yourself eating before hunger strikes. If you over- or under-eat one evening, note how long it takes for your appetite to return the following morning.

2. Write down your most common thoughts about food and exercise. Place a checkmark next to the items that empower metabolism, and put an X beside the ones that drain you. Replace the draining statements with empowering ones.

3. Reevaluate your exercise and eating activities. Eliminate activities driven by fear, resentment, or anger, and replace them with activities driven by inspiration.

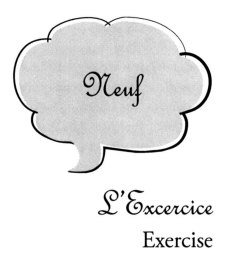

L'Excercice
Exercise

The true purpose of exercise is to invigorate and strengthen us in body, mind and spirit.
—Deepak Chopra, "Overcoming Addictions"

John and I greeted each day in Paris with a modest breakfast of yogurt, fruit, muesli, and coffee in the hotel café, followed by a vigorous walk to the neighborhood park. Once we arrived at our destination, we eased into our morning run, beginning with a light jog and then working up to a brisker pace worthy of our self-images as serious fitness people.

Soon we noticed that we were the only *runners*. The locals walked the park or, better said, strolled the park. So rather than appear to be escaping a crime scene, we worked on blending in. Even so, our brisk walking pace really didn't match the leisurely tempo set by the strikingly fit-looking locals. We still came across as frantic Americans—there was no way around that.

So we started to walk more slowly. The idea of consuming all that delicious French fare *and* disregarding the mathematics of calories in versus calories out caused us a bit of anxiety. But hey, this was a vacation, after all, and when in Paris . . .

Now that we were in a more reflective mood, we occasionally stopped to take notice of the places throughout the park where bars had been installed that appeared to be specifically designed for extending the limbs. At these stations, people engaged in general, deliberate, feel-good stretching. Not stretches that preceded or followed exertion—just stretching for the all-over relaxing and invigorating effect. This was not at all the obligatory activity that we were accustomed to engaging in after a run, for example. The stretching we observed in Paris *was the exercise*. A lot of strollers and a lot of stretchers—that's what I noticed as the ninth secret took form in my mind: Moderate exercise is all the body really needs.

According to clinical psychologist Eliezer Margoles, PhD, who seems to agree with the French philosophy, feeling joyful and experiencing the pleasure of being in one's body is very beneficial. He cautions against a "punitive" mind-set in which exercise is a task or even a punishment.* Instead, he wants us to find pleasure in movement, to feel it as something positive and a way to maintain wellness—and not just physical wellness, but mental wellness.

And we didn't see one gym in all of France. I'm sure they were there—perhaps tucked in the bowels of the American hotels to accommodate American travelers. It seemed that the French took their exercise as a way of saluting the day—by moving a little outdoors, but certainly not breaking a sweat.

One of the highlights of our morning walk was passing the schoolyard at recess. Each morning we listened for the bell of freedom and watched the swarms of children pour out of the schoolhouse. They ran and jumped and laughed until they reached their chosen destination. Some hit the grass and played marbles; others just ran and ran in circles through the park. In uniform but not at all restricted, they seized the beauty of the moment.

Even more compelling than the visual image was the sound—the clatter of happy children laughing, talking, screaming. The last time I heard children laughing and screaming here in the States I was with a group of women standing near a school playground. "What's that *noise?*" one of the women asked. "It's sure *irritating*," another commented.

Clotilde Dusoulier explains, "Many of us in France lead naturally active lives, especially in cities, running this way and that using our feet and public transportation to go around because a car would just get you stuck in traffic: I myself walk for forty minutes every day just to go to and from work, and there are tons of stairs in the metro."

Requia Badr was raised in Paris starting at the age of five and publishes the blog *Chez Requia: Cuisine et Confidence*. She adds, "We walk quite a lot compared maybe to some cities in the U.S. I remember the day I was walking on Third Street in Los Angeles and three different cars stopped and the drivers asked, 'What happened? Are you okay?' This couldn't occur in France because we are accustomed to walking. When I can avoid taking the bus or the metro I do it, and anyway, even taking the metro, we walk a lot from one line to another."

Estelle Tracy shares her perspective on exercise: "I do not exercise much, but I try and walk every day around lunchtime. Besides, I do vacuum at home. If you are not convinced it is exercise, feel free to show up at my place and clean all the rooms!"

Deprivation Nation

In grade school I couldn't wait for physical education class; I loved to run and participate in any activity presented. I was naturally athletic. It was something I never really thought about, like breathing—until one day our P.E. teacher told us that we would be working toward something called the Presidential Physical Fitness Award.

I really didn't think twice about it——as long as there was something physical going on, I was happy. One of the five events was a pull-up exercise. The idea was to pull your chin above the parallel bar using your arms for strength while steadily hanging on, keeping your chin above the bar, of course. And hang on I did, and on, and on and on . . . until I heard my classmates screaming and jumping and cheering me on. My P.E. teacher shouted out the seconds from the official stopwatch as the kids screamed louder and louder.

Apparently I'd broken a record. I really didn't get it. I could have hung there like a monkey in my bright blue gym frock all morning, and apparently I did for quite some time. It reminds me of the times I make a fuss over my dogs' most basic moves, and they look at me, confused, as if to say. "I don't get it. I just did a normal dog thing—what's the big deal?"

Anyway, I won the Presidential Physical Fitness Award. It was a big deal at my school and a defining moment for me. The award recognizes students who achieve an outstanding level of physical fitness. You must score on or above the 85th percentile on all five events to receive the award. I remain amused by receiving an award for something that was so *natural*.

Where along the way did tyrannical exercise routines replace the joy, the fun, and the natural? In my case it was in 1994, when I met my first personal trainer, Meri.

I was in a demanding career, working long hours, and my thinking was that some physical activity would help balance the stress. I contacted Meri based on the recommendation of a friend, and we met in the gym soon after.

A sweet little Southern girl with wild bleached-blonde hair was not what I had expected, and the sweetness lasted only until our first session began. Jillian Michaels has nothing on Meri—*nothing*. A lawyer turned personal trainer, she was as serious as could be about the work she was doing; in fact, she was obsessive.

My first assignment was to show up two days later at 5:15 A.M., ready to "train"—whatever that meant. I was also instructed to bring along a food journal, noting everything I had consumed in the interim. I did what anyone with a firing brain cell would do—I cleaned up my act. Out with the white chocolate scones from the Corner Café, in with the raisin bran.

"She'll be impressed with my food choices," I thought to myself.

Impressed she was not. She had a fit. "*Raisin bran?*" she shouted, "Are you kidding me? Do you know how many carbs are in *raisin bran?*"

"Uh—no, not really . . . I never thought about it," I confessed.

She turned on her heels (no easy feat, since she was wearing clogs), her ratted-up, bird's-nest of a bleached-blonde hairdo flying behind her, and returned with a stack of papers. "Here is your plan," she said firmly. "Stick to this. You can cheat one day a week—that's it."

"And here are some recipes. I'll give you a few each week," she instructed. The rest of the session is a blur in my memory—after all, it began at 5:15—but I'm sure it went well beyond an hour. Meri had a mission. It wasn't about her hourly rate; it was about sculpting and controlling me into submission.

For the next month or so I fell asleep at my desk around 3:00 P.M. on the three days a week that I trained with Meri. My muscles ached constantly, and I was always hungry. But a commitment is a commitment, and I was determined to see it through.

I'd never before in my life followed a diet—this was brand-new territory. I decided not to take the cheat day, thinking it would only make things worse. And as I mentioned, I'm no punk. Remember: I earned the Presidential Award for Physical Fitness.

I became the teacher's pet, doing everything just as Meri ordered—and sometimes even going beyond the call. And I liked her; I really liked her. You can get pretty close to a person when you spend time with them before dawn three days a week.

Before long I was a sculpted specimen. Meri was proud. "Wear a sleeveless dress to the party," she insisted. "I want everyone to see your arms."

And so I did. I received a lot of positive comments at first, but before long my friends were commenting that maybe it was time to cool it a little. I had never been overweight, and as my friend Donna was honest enough to tell me, "You look like a lollipop with a big head and a stick body."

I'm not sure what kept me going on this punishing regimen. Was it the ability, in the face of a life in which I was pushed this way and that by a demanding schedule, to control *something* myself, or the desire to please Meri, or maybe even both?

Either way, for more than two years I continued the sessions with Meri. "You seem to enjoy deprivation," my pal John commented between bites during lunch. "You actually make it look easy."

Deprivation? What was he talking about? Maybe I didn't understand him correctly with that evil chocolate cake in his mouth.

We are a nation of obsessive exercise "junkies" who experience the same withdrawal symptoms as heroin addicts when they try to stop, with medical findings to prove it. Cooling it when it comes to exercise gives new meaning to the term "cold turkey." Experts are telling us that withdrawal systems are similar in exercise fanatics and drug addicts.

An exercise program usually starts innocently enough with a desire for health and fitness but can easily become an obsession as alluring as taking narcotics— running distances that are too long, lifting weights that are too heavy, too many days in the gym each week—especially when the exercise is motivated by a desire to lose weight and keep it off.

(Before you take this as the perfect excuse to remain in that comfy corner of your living room couch, keep in mind that the lead researcher whose study on addictive exercise was published in the journal *Behavioral Neuroscience,* also noted: "As with food intake and other parts of life, moderation seems to be the key. . . . Exercise, as long as it doesn't interfere with other aspects of one's life, is a good thing with respect to both physical and mental health."*)

I'm not sure when exactly I tired of the routine, but I do remember that as a bridesmaid at my friend's wedding I finally caved for a piece of wedding cake. I figured it was my duty. Afterward I felt guilty, a failure, for leaving my plan in the dust along with the cake crumbs. Yet my instincts were keen enough to know that limiting carbohydrates for two years couldn't possibly be good for my health.

So I continued training with Meri but adapted my plan to something a little more balanced and also began my studies in nutrition. After a year of reading nutritional material for pleasure, I decided to go back to school for a degree in holistic nutrition.

Staring Down a Wolf in Sheep's Clothing

In order to unravel my unbalanced behavior, I studied with great interest, eagerly learning the many ways in which whole foods support the body and health in general. I always had a genuine respect for my health and physical welfare—never, for example, smoking or drinking—so studying nutrition was a way for me to raise the bar. My new eating plan fell under the category of "healthy eating" and allowed me to exist within a larger and slightly more flexible box.

Of course, the foods I named unhealthy were out of the question, so my control mechanism was intact. I pursued dietary purity and wellness through "healthy eating" habits and felt clearheaded and enlightened.

Little did I know at the time about a preoccupation called *orthorexia*, the term for an obsession with eating only healthy foods. Though it is motivated by a desire to feel healthy, natural, and pure—as opposed to anorexia, a desire to lose weight—it is nonetheless a disorder that has taken over the lives of many afflicted individuals. It is the "wolf in sheep's clothing" of eating disorders. I may not have known about orthorexia at the time, but I did know that the sweetness of life disappeared with my fixation on eating only healthy food. I eventually decided it was better to eat pizza with friends than to eat tofu, brown rice, and adzuki beans alone.

By the beginning of the year 2000, I had earned my degree and set up a private practice in Atlanta. Meri became not only a client but also one of my biggest supporters. I can thank her for playing a major role in building my practice of more than three hundred clients. By this time Meri owned her own gym and believed that the nutritional component would ensure the success of our mutual clients. It was a good plan for all concerned. It was also good that Meri was out of the business of offering extreme diet programs. And I was eating carbs again, albeit "healthy" carbs.

For the next couple of years I concentrated on building my private practice. I employed a private chef, engaged in some public speaking, and wrote nutritional articles for a few local publications. I worked with two professional athletes and a couple of high-profile clients. My work was very gratifying and at the same time enlightening.

I saw that adopting self-sabotaging habits around food was common, especially emotional eating. Often I didn't feel equipped to handle the complexity of these deep-rooted issues, and I found myself referring many of my clients to trusted psychotherapists.

It was important to me that I provide a good example for my clients. Even though I had a much more balanced approach to eating than many of them did, I still had my "rules," which fell more or less under the umbrella of "healthy eating." I didn't allow myself much in the way of decadence, that's for sure. It took me a while to understand that by allowing myself to be human, I would actually be a better example, as well as a more realistic and effective nutritional consultant.

I also had a great vantage point from which to observe other people's strategies for managing their weight. I saw the way a client would tighten the noose after she had a little success, just as I had done. It was not the least bit unusual to have a client state, for example, "Two years ago I had a lot of success on the South Beach diet." I would respond, "Well, exactly how do you define success?"

The answer would normally be that she had lost weight—that was success. I would point out that now she had gained back the weight and was in my office looking for another diet, another program, another silver bullet. Usually my client took the rap, blamed herself for a lack of willpower, and vowed not to mess up again. Yet, she still wanted a diet. "Just give me the plan, and I'll follow it this time" was something I heard way more than once.

That's when I had my first revelation—there is no *one* plan. With weight management, one size does not fit all. *On est individualiste!* So beginning with myself, I designed a hybrid way of eating dictated by my palate alone, my unique heritage, my lifestyle. Most important, my way of eating was health-supportive but also left room for the pleasure that food is designed to deliver. I threw the whip in the trash bin with the diet books.

Remarkably, the same shift took place simultaneously in my personal life. I found that I was no longer concerned about the opinions of others regarding my life, but that I now cared very deeply about being true to myself. What a surprise to learn that the others I was so anxious about were all wrapped up in their own chaos and thought very little about what I was doing!

So, first, I administered some self-prescribed truth serum, as needed. Next, I shone a very bright light on the dark areas in my life, confronting toxic relationships and habits that I hadn't had the courage or time to illuminate while I was fixated on controlling my food rituals.

The best way I can describe the next phase of my life is this: It was like approaching a high dive wearing a blindfold, knowing that I must jump, but with the faith that I would hit cool, refreshing, cleansing water, rather than smack and splat all over an empty concrete pool.

Guess what? I swam like a fish! A very happy, free fish that had found the most comfortable body of water it had ever navigated.

From that very day forward my life flourished. I married my husband, John, twenty-six years after meeting him—yes, twenty-six years after discovering that he was the *one*. (Our story is another book altogether.)

That was some potent truth serum I was taking! Our trip to Paris was a dream come true. From the day I stood on the avenue de l'Opéra with my buddy Mark, I had dreamed of sharing my love of France with John. And, of course, in my newfound honest and true frame of mind, my disordered dieting and denial finally behind me, I was able to take in all that the experience had to offer.

Slim without the Gym

Randy was my trainer when we lived full-time in central Florida. I'd come a long way from the days of Meri the militant. Randy was a fun-loving guy who worked out when he felt like it. Quite a comic and very entertaining, he was always amusing to be around. Often I didn't quite work up a sweat, but I had some deep belly laughs, especially when Randy broke out in a Tim McGraw–like serenade of "Seventeen."

For a short time John and I lived in Las Vegas, an experience that was quite surreal. At the time I was running regularly—maybe five miles a day—and my running trail became the Las Vegas strip. Talk about eye candy! There was no need for an iPod—music blasts everywhere—and the billboards and lights provide constant entertainment. I ran up and down the steps, crossing the street and back again. I ran through hotel lobbies and out again. I've never enjoyed running more. To the night owls coddling their coffee like little moles peeking at the breaking day, I must have seemed like a crazy person. Sometimes they would even startle and jump when I sped by!

I decided that I needed to cross-train, so I contacted a trainer referred to me by the fitness center at Trump Towers. I phoned Jeff, a "celebrity" trainer, and during an introductory phone call we hit it off immediately. I was eager to meet him in person. He told me to take a look at *Las Vegas* magazine, which was running an article featuring him. I happened to have the magazine on hand and opened it while we were on the phone. *Ooh la la!* Jeff had muscle where I didn't know humans even *have* muscles. I said, "Okay, you'll do—I guess."

It turned out that Jeff is a model as well, a big-time model—for Versace, Polo, Nike, to name a few—with the good looks to prove it. All of a sudden my husband,

John, took an interest in training. We had a lot of fun working with Jeff, who is sort of like a really good-looking, extremely fit Tony Robbins—optimistic and passionate about life.

The twenty-four-hour gyms in Vegas are fascinating—strippers, transvestites, cabana candy (girls paid to hang around the Vegas pools), show people, and the two of us. Jeff and I ran the strip occasionally, and he worked on helping me balance out my training regimen.

John and I and Jeff and his beautiful Brazilian wife, Priscila, became fast friends. Pri traveled most of the week on modeling assignments, so typically we got together to relax on Sunday. I soon observed that Pri was able to throw back a plate of ribs like a linebacker.

It's interesting watching her eat—she knows exactly what she has "a taste" for, and once she's had enough, that's it. She eats what she wants, when she wants it, until she is satisfied. Food is not a moral or emotional issue for her. She does not describe foods as good or bad; to her they are neutral, just food.

More than anything, Pri *savors* her food. Sometimes she rubs her belly and rolls her eyes back in satisfaction. At first, it all seemed very unusual behavior indeed for a swimsuit model, but the pieces of the puzzle were slowing fitting together for me.

A year later John and I lived for a while in Park City, Utah. Out in the cool crisp air, nestled among the mountain ranges that surrounded our home, I channeled my French experience. Oddly enough, Park City provided some vivid reminders of my time abroad. Open-air markets offered some of the best produce I have tasted in our country, and wonderful restaurants featured homemade breads almost as dense as the ones we enjoyed in Europe.

I thought about my foreign exchange student Bernie. While he was in the States he never found the kind of bread he had loved in Austria. I suspected the bread we ate in Utah would have come close. Without the distractions of a large city, I spent my mornings hiking with my dogs, my afternoons shopping in the markets, and evenings preparing meals. Immediately, John commented on the freshness of the ingredients, "Even salads just taste better," he marveled.

Jeff and Pri spent Thanksgiving with us in Park City. Following the big feast, we enjoyed leftovers for four days. Jeff encouraged us to "take the hill," and we walked and ran and played with the dogs on the mountain trails. There isn't a better place in the world for an elite athlete than Park City, Utah. Once you become accustomed to the altitude, you are able to enjoy the challenge of the topography as well as clean, crisp air that is void of any humidity.

No one could ever replace Jeff as far as I was concerned, and since the great outdoors offered so many natural opportunities for exercise I decided to forgo the gym and a personal trainer for the first time since 1994. For the next six months I walked the trails daily, thoroughly enjoying every movement. My exercise regimen was *natural* again—finally.

Eating what I wanted, when I wanted, trying to relax a bit, and moving rather than exercising—all of this required a big leap of faith. I guess I still thought there was something special in French "genetics" that accounted for the French figure. But by this time I willing to roll the dice . . . I remained calm, happy, and free—feelings that I'd buried for more than sixteen years. Life was *good*, and my clothes were loose!

Back in central Florida, "You look like you've lost weight," my hair stylist noticed. "And your arms look so toned. What are you doing?" she inquired.

I told her that I wasn't exercising much, just walking my dogs daily, eating normally.

"Okay, don't tell me your secret," she laughed.

"No, no, honestly, that's it," I insisted.

"You're not running anymore?" another stylist asked.

"Nope, just walking every day—I'm really enjoying it." This was followed by another a doubtful gaze—hmmm. Considering the bill of goods we have all been sold and the power we've given the dogma of dieting, I suppose skepticism was to be expected. *N'est-ce pas?*

Walk the Walk

Now that we live in New York City we've really stepped it up. John walks to and from his office every day—about 1.2 miles each way. In my daily errands, meetings, and activities, I'm sure I cover a minimum of 4 miles each day. This may be typical for New Yorkers living in the city, but it's not the norm for the rest of the nation.

Here's how Americans compare to others around the world, according to researchers at the University of Tennessee. We average just 5,117 steps per day, far fewer than people in Australia (9,695), Switzerland (9,650), and Japan (7,168).*

American men take more steps per day than women—5,340 versus 4,912. In addition, single people in the United States take significantly more steps per day (6,076) than those who are married (4,793) or widowed (3,394), according to data collected from 1,136 U.S. adults.

"The health benefits of walking are underappreciated. Even modest amounts of walking, if performed on a daily basis, can help to maintain a healthy body weight," lead author Dr. David R. Bassett Jr., of the University of Tennessee Obesity Research Center in Knoxville, said in an American College of Sports Medicine news release.

WALK YOUR WAY TO BETTER MEMORY
AND A STRONGER BRAIN

Exercise increases blood flow to your whole body, including your brain. Exercise seems to slow the loss of brain tissue that typically begins when people are in their forties. And exercise increases blood flow to a brain area involved in memory. No one knows the perfect exercise formula for brain health—some experts say 30 to 60 minutes, three times a week—but simply walking has shown benefits. A sharper brain makes a sexier dame!

Maybe this helps us to better understand why obesity rates are much higher in the United States than in other developed countries. Thirty-four percent of U.S. adults are obese, compared with 16 percent in Australia, 8 percent in Switzerland, and 3 percent in Japan.

"The results of our study are reasonably consistent with data from surveys of travel behavior," Bassett said. "In Switzerland and Japan, a much higher percentage of trips are taken by walking, compared to the United States. This is reflected in their greater daily step counts, and the additional walking seems to have an enormous public health benefit for those countries."

And yet another report on walking and health, published in 2010 in the *American Journal of Preventive Medicine*, showed that Americans who walked more than 5,000 steps a day were 40 percent less likely to develop metabolic syndrome—often a precursor to diabetes—and those who walked 10,000 or more steps were 72 percent less likely to develop it.*

Finally, I happen to be from Pittsburgh, so the news of a study done there recently that suggests that walking could actually prevent the brain from shrinking intrigued me.* The study suggests that nine miles a week is just about right for "neurological exercise." Just walking naturally—doing errands, getting from here to there—is a simple defense against dementia and Alzheimer's. "Our results should encourage well-designed trials of physical exercise in older adults as a promising approach for preventing dementia and Alzheimer's disease," said Dr. Kirk Erickson, of the University of Pittsburgh, who led the study. It's kind of a no-brainer. We can get smaller waistlines, maintain sharp brains, and avoid disease by doing something as easy as putting one foot in front of the other for half an hour a day.

Brittle Bones and Irregular Periods: Avoidable Risks

I learned recently through a dual energy X-ray absorptiometry (DXA) scan that my bone-mineral density is lower than normal, a condition called osteopenia.

Weight training builds stronger bones and muscles, so what about all of the years I spent in the gym? Isn't that exactly what it takes to maintain healthy bones? The answer is yes—*but in balance*. My muscles were so lean that for more than eighteen months at the height of my training I experienced menstrual interruptions due to my lack of adequate body fat. That interruption could in part be responsible for my thinning bone today.

CORRECTING THE MYTHS BEHIND OSTEOPOROSIS

Osteoporosis Is Not	*Osteoporosis Is*
Just thin bones	Thin and substandard bone
Common all over the world	Common only in Westernized countries
Normal and the result of aging	A degenerative disease
A female disorder	A feminist issue in Westernized countries
A disorder of the elderly	Common among the young
An isolated disorder	A manifestation of systemic breakdown
Something that goes wrong with bones	A bodily response to long-term imbalance

I now know that excessive exercise and an inadequate diet (such as my dairy-free phase) can lead to long-term menstrual irregularities, known as *amenorrhea*. Amenorrhea can result in low bone density at multiple skeletal sites, especially the spine.

In a misguided effort to be lean and healthy, I may have contributed to a condition that strikes many apparently vigorous female athletes and dancers. In addition to low bone density, amenorrhea can also affect a woman's fertility.

Fortunately, my thinning bone is occurring in my right hip and not yet in my spine, and my bone density is not low enough to be classified as osteoporosis. But it could be if I don't work to rebuild the thinning bone. I eat a good amount of foods rich in calcium and supplement daily with calcium and vitamin D.

Osteoporosis affects 25 million Americans, mostly women, and the majority of women don't know it until a fall results in a broken bone. A doctor might also make a diagnosis when a patient scores significantly below normal on a bone density test.

Another sign is diminished height. People don't get shorter as they get older because of bad posture. What actually happens is that fragile, osteoporotic vertebrae collapse and the spine compresses.

My mother, who is now ninety-three, probably started losing bone in her forties. Only recently, when she fell and broke her hip, did we discover she had osteoporosis. Each year more than 300,000 people end up in the hospital with hip fractures due to osteoporosis. Half of these people never go home again, and one in five dies from complications within a year. Even if she is lucky enough to survive and doesn't end up in a nursing home, a woman who has broken a hip or even a wrist may lose her independence because she's so fearful of falling again.

PRACTICING YOUR FRENCH

This week:

1. Visit the local playground. Swing on the swing, throw a ball, jump rope—whatever brings you the joy you remember as a child. *This* is exercise.

2. The next time you exercise, be honest—do you derive pleasure from this activity, or are you whipping yourself into submission? If you are not fully engaged in pleasure, switch it up until you find just the right activity.

Interlude
Adieu Hershey

FOR THOSE OF US WHO have joined the cult of *le chocolat*, chocolate emporiums and online boutiques are popping up everywhere—including websites from several of the Parisian chocolatiers listed below.

When You're in France . . .

If you're a chocolate lover, you can indulge that attraction along with your passion for Paris the next time you happen to be in France. The Paris Chocolate and Pastry Food Tour features French gourmet specialties as highlights of an afternoon walking tour of no more than eight people.

A food connoisseur will take you through a number of Paris neighborhoods to visit at least three pastry shops, a bakery, and three chocolate shops, including La Maison du Chocolat. For scheduling and pricing, visit www.viator.com and enter Paris Chocolate and Pastry Tour in the search field.

Listed below are at least one location for some of the best chocolatiers in Paris:

Patrick Roger
108 blvd. St-Germain – 75006 Paris

Named best French artisan in 2000, Patrick Roger is known for his *rochers* (smooth praline filling and crunchy hazelnut flecks), *ganaches* (chocolate and cream melted together), and dark chocolate complemented by flavors like lime or hot pepper. The original Patrick Roger store is in the south Paris suburb of Sceaux.

La Maison du Chocolat
225 rue du Faubourg St. Honoré – 75008 Paris

Founded in 1977 by Robert Linxe (once referred to as a "*ganache magician*"), La Maison du Chocolat has several stores in Paris. If you don't like bitter chocolate, this is your shop—La Maison du Chocolat never uses more than 65 percent cocoa in their confections. World-renowned for its *ganaches*, this shop also specializes in truffles, *mendiants* (slices of chocolate topped with dried fruit or nuts), and bars with fruit or herbal notes.

Michel Chaudun
149 rue de l'Université – 75007 Paris

The former head of La Maison du Chocolat, Michel Chaudun is one of the world's best artisan chocolatiers. Known for his whimsy as much as for his mastery of the classics, he offers everything from simple dark or milk bars and truffles to chocolates crafted to look exactly like sausages.

Christian Constant
37 rue d'Assas – 75006 Paris

Christian Constant has two shops in Paris, one close to the Luxemburg Gardens and the other near the Opera. His chocolate is rated by food critics as among the world's finest, and he gets high marks for delicacies like raspberry *ganaches*, chocolate-covered orange peel, chocolates with spicy or herbal notes, and his famous *palet d'or*, made from fresh cream and dark chocolate. Constant also offers cakes and pastries and five decadent varieties of hot chocolate.

Josephine Vannier
4 rue du Pas de la Mule – 75003 Paris

This jewel of an artisanal chocolate shop, in the Marais district on the Right Bank, offers a wide array of creations, from chocolate masks, mini-grand pianos, and all-chocolate replicas of vintage ads to classics like crispy *nougatine*, truffles, and *mendiants* (chocolate disks garnished with nuts, seeds, dried fruits, and other delicacies).

HOW TO ENJOY CHOCOLATE

As with all things French, but especially chocolate, favor quality over quantity. It takes several pieces of inferior milk chocolate to satisfy my sweet tooth, but only one piece of high-quality dark chocolate.

Keep chocolate at room temperature (65–72 degrees F). Too warm and it'll go soft; too chilly, and it won't melt properly and release flavor in your mouth in the way the maker intended.

The bar's surface should be free of blemishes, such as white marks (called bloom). The bloom is cocoa butter that has separated and risen to the surface, a result of improper storage and temperature changes that also make the chocolate lose its shine. Not to worry—it's still safe to eat and will taste fine. Even so, in good chocolate, the bar should show a radiant, glossy sheen.

The texture can be the most obvious clue about quality: Low-quality bars have a grainy, almost cement-like texture. Breaking a piece of high-quality chocolate results in a resounding *snap!* The broken edge will be fine, smooth, and glossy.

Smell the chocolate, especially at the break point. Inhaling the aroma primes your tongue and previews the nuances of the flavor. Place the chocolate on your tongue and let it melt. Chew it only to break it into small enough pieces that it begins to melt. Concentrate on the variety of flavors that are released. Enjoy this moment of bliss, and bask in the contentment that only chocolate imparts.

I eat a 1.6-ounce bar of good-quality dark chocolate every day. Dark chocolate's bitter taste helps the body regulate appetite; the high levels of cocoa butter help slow digestion and make the stomach feel full longer. For me, nothing short of this prescription for pleasure will keep off the pounds.

Michel Cluizel

201 rue St-Honoré – 75001 Paris

Michel Cluizel chocolates have been renowned since the middle of the twentieth century, when Cluizel first opened a family-run shop in Normandy. At this store near the Tuileries Gardens, visitors can indulge in delicious dark or milk bars and purchase whole cocoa beans, which can be roasted, then peeled, ground, and mixed with cinnamon and sugar to make hot chocolate.

Pierre Hermé

72 rue Bonaparte – 75006 Paris

Perhaps the world's most celebrated pastry chef, Pierre Hermé has also won rave reviews for his line of gourmet chocolates. The main shop in the St. Germain district offers an unparalleled selection of chocolate cakes, pastries, and *macarons*. Death by Chocolate consists of a moist chocolate biscuit base layered with smooth chocolate cream, frothy chocolate mousse, and fine leaves of crunchy chocolate.

. . . and When You're Not

What about when you're not in Paris? Instead, you're in the good old US of A and you're browsing in a local food shop that offers a display of chocolates that go beyond Hershey's and Cadbury. Look for products made by some of these great American chocolatiers; even some French brands can be purchased in specialty stores like one of my favorites—Valrhona. If you can't find specialty chocolates in your area, they are available online through sites like www.worldwidechocolate.com.

Guittard Chocolate Company

An experienced chocolate maker, Frenchman Etienne Guittard took along delicious French chocolate to trade for mining supplies when he joined the California Gold Rush in the 1850s and discovered that wealthy miners would pay premium prices for this elegant treat. When he returned to France, Guittard worked in his uncle's chocolate factory until he could afford to buy his own chocolate-making equipment. In 1868 he opened Guittard Chocolate on San Francisco's Sansome Street.

Ghirardelli Chocolate

America's longest continuously operating chocolate manufacturer (in business for more than 150 years), Ghirardelli offers rich, high-quality products by controlling the chocolate manufacturing process from cocoa bean to finished product.

Dagoba Organic Chocolate

Dagoba Organic Chocolate was founded in 2001 by Fredrick Schilling, whose mission was to organically produce a fine chocolate and infuse it with ingredients that would appeal to the adventuresome palate.

Scharffen Berger

In 1997 two long-time friends—Robert Steinberg, a retired doctor, and John Scharffen Berger, former owner of Scharffen Berger Wineries—perfected a new small-batch chocolate-making process and created a company that specializes in dark chocolate.

Vermont Nut Free Chocolate Company

Founded by the mother of a little boy with a peanut allergy, this company offers products that are completely safe for those with any tree nut or peanut allergy but that can also be enjoyed by anyone who loves fine chocolates. ✤

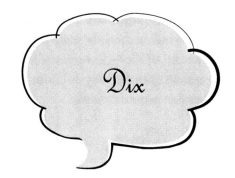

Dix

Les Rythmes et les Rituels
Rhythms and Rituals

As we share the breaking of bread . . . as we
share words, I am also breaking my life, I am
breaking open my memory and sharing
it with others, and they with me.
—Jean Molesky-Poz, former Franciscan monk

WHILE VISITING NEW ORLEANS after Hurricane Katrina I became acquainted with our tour director, a lifelong resident of the city—a woman who had lost her home in the devastation of the hurricane. We were seated together at lunch, and as we shared a whiskey bread pudding I asked her to describe the most significant events in her experience following the hurricane.

She thought for a few moments, took a deep breath, and described waking up in the middle of the night wondering what happened to the gentleman who played the harmonica on the corner every day as she waited for the bus. She had never known him by name, but he was an important part of her daily life. That was before Katrina—now he is gone and she is left wondering about his fate. I was reminded that we often take for granted the simple rhythms and rituals of our daily routine, yet they can frame our lives as firmly as the walls of the rooms we live in.

In France the rituals and rhythms of life are so transparent that I feel a little sheepish calling them the tenth secret. Empires may come and go, but in France the sacraments of life—pleasure, tradition, and *la cuisine*—are revered. It is impossible to examine the disparity in eating habits of our countries without observing the values that surround them.

Beyond Grocery-Store Donuts

One of my fondest memories and rituals began when I was a young girl sharing donuts with my father every Saturday morning. Among our favorites were the Sweet Sixteen brand of powdered-sugar and chocolate-coated delicacies. We were dunkers and dipped our donuts in strong coffee until they were fully saturated and just right. I always ended up with lots of powdered sugar on my face, my lips and fingertips, my coffee cup, and the table. My father was a man of few words, and we often spent time together not saying much of anything. Even so, there was more meaning in the ritual than a million words could express.

My father passed away on a Saturday. I called him several times that morning, wondering if he had already picked up the donuts or whether I should grab them on the way over. He never answered my call. I can't look at a Sweet Sixteen donut bag without remembering him.

For many years following my father's death I didn't eat a donut; initially I just couldn't bear it, and then of course donuts weren't exactly on my diet plan.

One afternoon when I was feeling melancholy and a bit lonely I grabbed a bag of powdered-sugar and chocolate-covered Sweet Sixteens. I guess on some level I expected to find my father among the sixteen donuts and hoped to bring some sweetness back into my life.

I started with the chocolate-covered . . . they were horrible—really horrible. The chocolate coating tasted like wax. I had another one just to be sure—same thing: wax. Then I tasted the powdered-sugar donut—better, but not really great. I was eating the food of a twelve-year-old. Somehow I had outgrown Sweet Sixteen donuts. I gave up on finding anything other than grocery-store donuts in the bag.

Many years later I was in New Orleans and, like many other visitors to the French Quarter, found myself at the famous French Market Café du Monde, on Decatur Street. You must have the beignets at the Café du Monde, and you certainly must dunk them in the café au lait.

And guess what? Powdered sugar everywhere—just like when I was a kid. Without any effort or idea of what memories this would evoke, I called to mind my father and dreamed that he was with me, not saying much of anything but dunking his beignet until it was just right, as we had always done. It was our ritual, and I'll never forget it.

"What's a ritual, anyway?"

Rituals are treasured traditions that we repeat over time. A common ritual is the reading of a bedtime story as you tuck your little ones in for the night. Rituals create warm, nurturing bonding experiences and offer the comfort of belonging. They can impart a sense of wonder, magic, and celebration to holidays and other special occasions.

Rituals help hold families together and move us emotionally from one place to another. They ease pain, acknowledge growth, and create connection. Rituals reinforce values.

Rather than try to discourage distractions that might shift the focus from the enjoyment of a meal, the French take a more proactive, positive approach that promotes dining rituals—such as serving three-course meals and using real plates and napkins—that are ingrained in the French tradition of *les arts de la table*. When asked about eating in front of the TV, Requia Badr explained:

> Actually, during the week, dinner is the only moment I can eat together at home with my husband. We always set the table with nice plates, napkins, etc., and we try to make time to enjoy dinner. It's really important to make time for dinner instead of eating in a few minutes and watching TV for the whole evening after. These rituals are really important because once again it's the only moment during the day when we can really communicate, and I don't think this can be possible if the TV is switched on. We can also really appreciate our dinner, appreciate what we cooked. These rituals are also important to me because at home with my parents dinner was an important moment. All the family was gathered round the table.

"I think my main focus is to make my environment as pleasant as I can before I start eating, so I can properly enjoy my meal," Clotilde Dusoulier says.

> I make sure I am comfortably seated in a nice atmosphere, with everything I'm going to need on hand—silverware, water, condiments, napkin. And I have no rule whatsoever against doing something else while I eat. In fact, I am usually doing something else

while I eat, whether it's talking to my dining companion(s), reading a book or a magazine if I'm alone, or even (gasp!) watching TV or a DVD—as long as it's something I (or we) truly enjoy.

My favorite way of spending an evening on my own is to eat a carefully home-cooked dinner for one, while watching *Sex in the City*. And a little chocolate rounds this out beautifully. In my opinion this just heightens the pleasure of the moment, and it doesn't draw my attention away from the food—but I'll admit that drawing my attention away from the food does take quite a lot!

At one point I was discussing this book with my mother, and she asked, "What's a ritual, anyway?"

"You pray before each meal," I reminded her. "That's a ritual, Mom. You bow your head in thanksgiving for the food before you, in respect for those who have farmed and prepared the nourishment you about to digest."

We don't stop to think about some of the most important rituals in our lives. The sacrament of prayer is one of great wisdom. It sanctions our slowing down and thus assists the body in the processes of assimilation and digestion—just another example of the power of prayer.

Simply stated, rituals are all about honoring time, taking time. You've heard the old saying "Time is money." In this case, the old saying is not true. Time is not money. Time is life, and it can't be enjoyed without slowing down.

A Personal Tradition—And It's Not Even French!

Everything you see I owe to spaghetti.

—Sophia Loren

My mother makes the best rigatoni and meatballs in the world. I know, I know: All Italians thinks their mother makes the very best tomato sauce, but I'm telling you—*mine does.*

Over the years my mother has been tempted to tweak the family sauce. Once, influenced by an Italian friend, she added crushed tomatoes and bay leaf. I had a fit. "Don't alter the sauce," I begged. "It's perfect the way it is!" My cousin Trish said the same thing, and ultimately my mother agreed.

We beg for "rigs," and at ninety-three my mother continues to deliver the family favorite. My husband always overeats the "sewer pipes," our nickname for rigatoni, filling his plate two, sometimes three times. And who can blame him? It's delicious!

It has taken me years to perfect Mom's tomato paste–based delight, and during that time I've realized that it's the preparation of the sauce, the stirring and the anticipating, as much as the flavorful outcome that is so special. Mom's sauce brings on priceless feelings that only a lifelong ritual can deliver.

I've moved all around the country, and I've developed a moving-day ritual that makes my new home feel as if I've lived there forever. I write "IMPORTANT! TAKE TO KITCHEN AND UNPACK IMMEDIATELY!" in large letters with a black Sharpie, ensuring that the box containing everything I need to make a rigatoni dinner—cans of tomato paste, two large pots (one for the pasta, one for the sauce), a large colander for draining—arrives in the kitchen and is right there. After I make a quick trip to the supermarket for the fresh essentials, my sauce bubbles away for the rest of the day while I unpack. The aroma of the sauce fills our new nest. Wiping our chins the first evening in our new home, among boxes and chaos, we can say, "Home Sweet Home."

Your family already has its own traditions, which might be anything from Sunday morning pancakes to observing holidays in a certain way to a special place you always go for summer vacation. The way you celebrate birthdays or observe other special days, the way you say good-bye to each other every morning or shop for school clothes each year—all are the bits and pieces of which lives and memories are made.

Creating new mealtime traditions that work for your family is a simple matter. Try something new, and if you like it, repeat it. Eventually, that tradition will take on a life of its own and will become a sustaining part of your family's culture.

Les Trucs

So what's an American girl to do? How can we *Frenchify* (yes, it's a new word!) our lives? Living in an environment of American excess and speedy ways of doing everything makes it a bit more difficult to cultivate a French way of being.

It's not unlike, as we've seen, what happens to those who relocate to the United States from other countries and quickly adapt to larger portions and gain larger appetites (and waistlines).

We know that the French tend to avoid processed foods, that they stick to three meals a day, and that they strive to maintain a balanced diet. But do French women have a system of *trucs* (a collection of well-honed "tricks") that keep them thin? What rhythms do they follow as they go about their days?

"I'm not sure if these qualify as *trucs*, but here are a few rules I try to stick to (with exceptions, of course)," Clotilde Dusoulier discloses:

I make sure I eat vegetables at every meal (potatoes don't count!) and fruit for breakfast.

After a nice (read: plentiful) meal, I wait for the feeling of hunger to come back before I eat again, and I generally try to avoid eating just because it's time.

I read the labels on the things I buy and stick to foods that are good quality and not too processed—I stick to what I would call real food.

I keep enough ingredients on hand to whip up a quick and healthy meal, so that if I am very hungry there's always an easy but good-for-you option.

I rarely bake without a special occasion, when I have friends to help me eat whatever it is I've baked.

When I plan a meal for a dinner party, if one of the courses is rich, the other two will be light(er).

I don't eat a cookie/cake/pastry just because it's there. I figure if I'm going to eat that kind of thing, it's going to be the freshest I can find.

Requia Badr offers her *trucs*: "As far as I'm concerned, I try to eat everything I like and to compensate for this pleasure. Looking at my eating habits and looking at the people around me, especially at work (I work in the fashion field) the main *trucs* are the following."

We try to eat at regular time, and we try to avoid snacking between meals. Sometimes we just don't have time for a correct lunch because of a huge amount of work, but anyway we try to eat good products instead of sandwiches or fast food. In Paris, we can find more and more sort of healthy fast foods like at Cojean, a new fast-food restaurant where the design is very trendy, very Zen, and quite minimalist.

Talking about grocery stores, I think the other *truc* is also that we cook quite often to better control our food, to eat good food, and to have a real meal in the evening if we didn't eat so well during the day.

For me the main truc is that we also drink a lot of water instead of sodas. In France, we are very fond of mineral water, and we can find a lot of different types in the stores. By the way, in Paris we can also find water bars in some trendy shops. More and more different kind of waters are launched every year, maybe to face a high demand for these products. If I can give an example to illustrate this, it can

AN AMERICAN IN PARIS: FASHION AND STYLE

"The French also know how to dress!" Susan began. "I have always been a dress and skirt kind of gal and have a passion for scarves. I loved looking at the way French women accessorize. It's an art form!

"They wear the same suit every day but change it up with a scarf, shoes, and a handbag. Those three items are the most important part of a French woman's wardrobe," she went on to reveal. "And the clothing is always of good quality. Storage is an issue, you know. Back in the day, closets were considered a room, so space is scarce. That's why there are so many armoires."

When Susan told me about the first day of spring in Paris, I was captivated. "It's almost as if there's a secret memo that goes out to all the women in Paris. You head out one morning and the dark winter tights have disappeared, and all of the women are baring naked legs," she laughed! "I admire the way the French women, whatever their age, show off their greatest asset, whether it's beautiful legs in a short skirt or their smooth décolletage in a plunging neckline!

"Then in August, the stores close down for the entire month while the French hit the beach or some fabulous destination. They know when to stop and recharge," she added.

"Beauty is everywhere in France," Susan remembered fondly. "From the flower boxes on the windowsills to the architecture to presentation chocolates and cleverly decorated storefront windows.

"I feel that the French perceive beauty more intuitively than Americans—simply and individually," she explained. "Men love women of all ages, and young men appreciate the beauty of mature women. French women carry themselves with grace and beauty in a natural and carefree way. Yes, they are dressed nicely, but they are never heavily made up. They are chic and self-assured.

"They do believe in taking care of their skin, and many get facials at least twice a month," Susan added.

be this one: My best friend lives in the U.S. If she wakes up at 3 a.m. and can't sleep anymore, she used to go to the fridge, take out a giant ice-cream carton, and have some in front of the TV. In the same circumstance, I'll have a glass of fresh water!

Estelle Tracy admits: "Oh, yes, I have a whole set of rules that I try and stick to, and hopefully people won't think I torture myself after reading them."

First, I would like to mention that I don't forbid myself from eating any kinds of foods, unlike people on diets. I allow myself to have pastries and chocolate in reasonable quantities, since I have noticed that when "naughty" foods are permitted, you crave them much less.

Like Clotilde, I have three meals a day, and I usually have dinner with my husband, preferably not in front of the TV! I rarely snack, unless I am really hungry. If I do, usually in the mid-morning or around 4 p.m.—the time for *le goûter* in France—I eat a piece of fruit or drink a big cup of tea, in order to feel full and last until lunch or dinner. I often eat at the same time every day. Unlike most Americans, my husband and I have a relatively late dinner, around 7:30 or 8:00 p.m. I don't like the idea of having dinner too early, as you may be hungry before going to bed. However, I try not to eat anything within two hours before going to bed. One thing I should point out is that my husband is a small eater, so I am never tempted too much at a meal.

I stick to my rules pretty closely on weekdays, but I am a little more relaxed on weekends. Also, when I go to a restaurant, I try not to be the soup and salad kind of diner. I want to treat myself and enjoy a good meal that I won't be able to make at home. Although my parents always encouraged me to finish my plate when I was a kid, I rarely try to finish it in American restaurants, where portions are much bigger.

My *Trucs*

When I summoned my inner French girl, my initial *truc* was eating anything I desired—but only half the portion I was accustomed to. Soon I learned that half was just about right. Some of my other *trucs* are:

I dine with a linen napkin and my best china, and I garnish the plate, even when I'm eating alone.

Regardless of the time and effort it takes, I prepare a real meal from scratch.

I walk. Every day I take my dogs on a three-mile pleasure walk—rain or shine, sleet or snow. It may be exercise, but it feels like fun. I have not been inside a gym in more than a year. I prefer to begin my day outdoors.

By eating smaller courses, I save room for dessert. I stay away from those loaded with refined sugar and hold out for homemade specialties. French desserts seem to be less sticky sweet. I visit my local French bakery once a week for my favorite—*tarte aux fruits.*

When I feel the urge to rush my meal and gulp my food, I pretend that I am being watched as I eat. This way I'm more likely to eat like a "lady."

Vegetables anchor my meals and account for at least 80 percent of the plate. I rarely eat meat; instead I choose fish, beans, and nuts. If I have a craving for a burger, I most certainly will indulge and usually can talk my husband into having one so that I can have a taste. Generally a bite or two satisfies my desire.

Water is my beverage of choice, although I do enjoy coffee in the morning. I've never been fond of alcohol; I can count on one hand the glasses of wine I've consumed in the last five years.

I eat a modest breakfast. Lunch is my main meal. I look forward to *le goûter*, something sweet or a piece of fruit and a slice of cheese. On days when I'm just not hungry in the afternoon, I skip the snack. Dinner is a lighter meal than lunch.

Fast food, processed food, and frozen food are of no interest to me. I would rather be hungry than eat inferior foods. I wait for the very best nourishment available.

Olive oil, avocado, nuts, and peanut butter are among my food staples. Add to that some wonderful bread or rolls, a great French jam, and an imported cheese, and I have everything I need!

If it doesn't taste good to me when it first passes my lips, I don't eat it or drink it, no matter what health benefits it promises.

When I shop, I strive for the very best options, but I'm not a fanatic. If I can't locate an organic item, I simple wash the fruit or vegetable thoroughly in a veggie-wash bath solution. I believe that the stress over a perfect diet is more harmful than the culprits we try to avoid.

I do aim for local food, and luckily every Saturday morning we have a wonderful farmers' market in our area where I am able to find fresh, organic, and local produce.

My Beauty *Truc*

Here's a beauty *truc* I had heard described in school and learned about in detail when I was in France—brushing your way to a cellulite-free beach body!

First, you'll need a body brush. Here in the United States, at the Body Shop (www.thebodyshop-usa.com) you can find a body brush that's much softer than the very firm brushes used in France—it's firm enough to do the job and quite a bit more pleasant. For best effects, I suggest you dry-brush yourself before you turn on the shower. Here's the routine I follow:

Start with a dry body and a dry brush, and begin with your feet. Give the soles of your tootsies a quick twirl, then brush from your toes right up over your ankles, and do the sides and backs of your feet the same way.

Brush in the longest strokes you can manage, up from your ankles to the tops of your legs. Go all around each leg with the long strokes. If your balance is too shaky to brush an entire leg at once, brush from your ankles to your knees, then from the knees to the tops of your thighs. I manage all of this just before showering, propping my foot on the bathroom vanity while watching the *Today* show.

Brush in additional long strokes from your thighs to your underarms. The long strokes are always upward; the aim is to brush toward the heart. Brushing your back is a bit awkward, so—if you're like me—you might want to cheat a little and use an old-fashioned back brush with a long handle.

Areas that tend to be more prone to cellulite—like the thighs, tummy, bum, and breasts—benefit from brisk circular brushing (go in one direction only, aiming to push toward the center of your body and upward)—then finish off with a couple more long, upward strokes.

Brush your hands and arms from your fingertips to your shoulders. Then you're finished. You can get through the whole process in about three minutes, though a French schoolgirl is expected to brush for ten minutes each morning!

Your brushing needs to be quite firm. Don't draw blood, but do aim to stimulate the circulation. Your skin will be pinkish red, and that's okay—a little evidence is healthy. You might feel tingly after your brushing. Brushing your skin can be quite addictive. Once you've dry-brushed for a few days, you don't feel clean after a shower without brushing first. My brush is always in my suitcase when I take a trip.

For an added touch of luxury, using my long-handled back brush (I don't like to get my smaller Body Shop, hand-held dry brush wet), I lather up with a bath gel, alternating between a relaxing lavender body gel and a revitalizing peppermint. To finish, I turn the temperature control to the coldest setting and wake up with a

INVEST IN YOURSELF

"Invest in yourself," my personal shopper, Ilsa, urged as I admired the singular pieces layered neatly on the table. The highly selective process of determining the key pieces of my basic wardrobe filled an entire afternoon. It's ten years later, and I still cherish the clothes I chose that day:

- A Dries Van Noten charcoal pinstriped pencil skirt tailored under Ilsa's careful scrutiny
- Black wool Jil Sander trousers, perfectly fitted
- Christian Louboutin high-heeled, animal print pumps
- The perfect black dress
- A Jil Sander charcoal velveteen riding coat
- Nude fishnet stockings
- A charcoal gray Jil Sander cashmere crew-neck sweater
- A chartreuse Jil Sander leather jacket

With Ilsa's help, I dressed to my strengths and my authenticity, selecting clothes that would endure decades of fads. I resisted the disposable, the trendy, and the faux. But more important than those practical decisions was the self-assurance I began to cultivate as I took the time to assess my life, my needs, and my comfort. Less was truly more. Instead of a closet full of not-so-great items, I chose just the right *quality* items for *me*. The values of quality, authenticity, evaluation, discretion, and self-possession, all very natural traits of the French girl, allowed me to engage in a custom-made life—a true reflection of myself.

I found my center that day and from that moment on embraced my individuality while resisting the pressure to be someone I'm not. I stopped taking shortcuts and said no to excess of all kinds. I uncovered my creativity in dressing—mixing and matching vintage items of extreme personal value with the basics Ilsa and I assembled.

The value of quality over quantity and all that this value holds is truly the main ingredient in living your best life, here or abroad.

blast of ice-cold water—and I'm good to go! It sounds like quite a process, but it's a wonderfully nurturing ritual that makes my day.

You'll need to replace the brush when the bristles look a bit sad—the same as with a toothbrush: as a rule, about once every six to eight weeks if you're using it daily. You'll notice visible results after about five months, and in the meantime you'll feel just great.

I first learned about the benefits of body brushing—stimulating circulation and exfoliation—when I was studying for my degree in holistic nutrition. After spending some time on the beaches of Cannes, I can attest to the advantages of body brushing in combating cellulite as well. But also remember that the diet of French women makes a big difference, too—plenty of water, fruits, and vegetables, and no processed foods!

L'hamburger, or Happy Meals in the Louvre

"Really, I'm not sure any woman in the world can eat and drink everything in large portions throughout the day without getting fat. If a woman can, she is really lucky!" Requia Badr articulates the rather obvious, if not disappointing reality from her home in Colombes, France.

The problem is that obesity is on the rise in France. Almost 20 percent of children are overweight, and the number classified as obese has more than doubled in ten years. It's a French dilemma.

So much for *French Women Don't Get Fat*. It's more like French women who don't pick up American values like fast food don't get fat. Not to mention the economic recession; it's no wonder that sales at France's 1,135 McDonald's outlets were up between 7 and 11 percent in 2009 over the previous year. As a matter of fact, the McDonald's on the avenue des Champs-Elysées continues to be the most profitable in the world.

Eating in McDonald's is almost a rite of passage for our young ones here in the United States. I can only hope that we don't share this American ritual to the point that it will sully the culinary legacy of the French.

Could it be that American tourists in France account for the traffic? Or are U.S.-driven globalization and American convenience starting to influence French culture? Are American eating habits spoiling ages-old (and healthy) French traditions? It seems it could be so, given the recent rise in obesity in France.

Now, much to the dismay of many a French citizen, a McDonald's has opened in the Louvre, downstairs in the food court among other fast-food outlets from around the world. Burt Hasqenof, who runs the website Louvre pour Tous (Louvre for All; louvrepourtous.fr), which keeps museum visitors informed about museum events and news, doesn't even consider McDonald's to be food: "It's based on the way to run a military organization," he said.

Is McDonald's a symbolic indication of a deeper problem? It seems that the museum was unable to veto McDonald's arrival since the Carrousel du Louvre, the food court, is operated by a private company, not the state-run museum. Commentators on louvrepourtous.fr are among those in France who have raised their eyebrows at the coming of McDonald's to the most French of French institutions, even in a food court that features cuisines of the world.

"Rendezvous in December for a Mona Lisa Extra Value Menu," Louvre Pour Tous wrote satirically, offering the challenge that the Louvre could have, and should have, put its foot down. Among all that we as Americans have to offer, is McDonald's the best we can come up with to represent what passes for American cuisine?

I don't know about you, but it offends me that the values of our nation are exploited and epitomized by an enterprise that favors low cost, large quantities, convenience, and impulsiveness over health and well-being.

PRACTICING YOUR FRENCH

This week:

1. Serve yogurt in a beautiful crystal bowl topped with fresh berries and nuts. Make the table beautiful, and eat your yogurt with a silver spoon.
2. Establish a family ritual based on a particular mealtime, special occasion, or celebration that you can commit to on a regular schedule. One idea might be a weekly build-your-own pizza night, followed by board games.
3. Read *The Book of New Family Traditions: How to Create Great Rituals for Holidays and Everyday*, by Meg Cox, for loads of mealtime ritual ideas.

Interlude
Red Wine, Flavonoids, and the Human Nervous System

I enjoy cooking with wine; sometimes I even put it in the food I'm cooking.

—Julia Child

"DRINK MORE WINE," the headlines of major U.S. newspapers boldly urged in the early 1990s.

The statistics don't lie: Despite their consumption of a significantly higher percentage of dietary fat per capita than Americans, the French boast lower blood cholesterol levels and heart disease. The intake of fat in the French diet would appear to be counteracted by their drinking of red wine. This line of thinking was bolstered by the fact that the intake of wine per capita in France was, at the time, higher than anywhere else in the world. In comparison, the U.S. per capita intake was among the lowest.

Researchers soon discovered that the chemical components in red wine called polyphenols—antioxidants that are present in the leaves, twigs, and bark of the grape vines, specifically a flavonoid called resveratrol—are the physical factor that provides a heart-protective effect. Yes, it *must* be the wine.

Next thing you know, scientists have isolated the polyphenols from wine, compounded them and squeezed them into resveratrol capsules, bottled them up, and *voilà*, they're available in every Walmart across the nation! Problem partially solved. At the same time, within four weeks of CBS's *60 Minutes* report (November 17, 1991) of the correlation between French consumption of red wine and heart disease, millions of Americans dash off to their local wine retailer. By mid-December 1991 sales of red wine increase by 44 percent in U.S. supermarkets.

But wait . . . Wine comes from grapes, so maybe it's not the alcohol in wine alone that accounts for the French Paradox. And if resveratrol is found not only in wine but also in the grapes that wine is made from, what about similar chemicals found in other fruits and vegetables? That, in fact, is where the research on the heart-protective effects of red wine have led—to the realization that foods, including grapes and wine, that contain polyphenols protect human health in a variety of ways (see in chapter 7, the section "A Paradox with a Payback," for more on polyphenols and the protections they afford).

The French habit of drinking a moderate amount of red wine with a meal is perhaps the best known (as in the most often discussed) contributor to the French Paradox, but I maintain that it is not the only or even the most fundamental contribution.

Yes, red wine is full of nutrients known to thin the blood and to lower blood pressure and bad cholesterol. However, this is true only when wine is absorbed in small doses and with food. Drinking too much alcohol without the benefit of greater absorption with food may be the difference between responsible alcohol use and irresponsible alcohol use and the potential for addiction.

The French view wine as a precious gift to be enjoyed, not abused. They do drink wine not to dull their senses but to awaken them to the enjoyment of food. Wine is always served with food in France. You will never see a French woman sipping a glass of Chardonnay as if it were a cocktail. The full taste of a wine is discovered only when it's paired with the right food.

So before you pop the cork, let's look at the bigger picture. In our typical American rush to bring to market a specific magic bullet (a pill, a glass or two of Merlot each evening), perhaps we're overlooking another, less quantifiable reason why the wine-drinking French have fewer strokes and heart attacks than we do. Maybe we are disregarding the unspoken effects of the physiological state of relaxation on maximum digestive function. Has anyone studied the effects of the parasympathetic nervous system on digestion and metabolic health?

Bear with me while I introduce a one-paragraph human biology lesson: The parasympathetic nervous system is the part of the autonomic (subconscious) nervous system that slows the heart rate, increases intestinal and gland activity, and relaxes the sphincter muscles. Sometimes referred to as the "rest and digest" system, it works in balance with the sympathetic nervous system, which accelerates the heart rate, constricts blood vessels, and raises blood pressure—physical processes that prepare us for the "flight or fight" response.

I believe that it's not the polyphenols in red wine alone that keep our French friends relatively free of heart disease. Their respect for and indulgence of the parasympathetic nervous system should also get kudos. The French deserve the credit for approaching the table in a peaceful, relaxed, joyful frame of mind that is, in fact, responsible for an optimum state of digestion and assimilation of nutrients.

One cannot bottle and sell values. Instead of focusing on the role of a single ingredient in the French diet, we would do better to cultivate the timeless, commonsense rituals of quality, respect, relaxation, balance, and pleasure each and every time we take a seat at the table. If that involves sipping a delicious wine along with some wonderful food, all the better. ❧

Les Valeurs
Values

To be blind is bad, but worse it
is to have eyes and not to see.
—Helen Keller

WHAT COULD BE a simpler secret than this one? Learn what you value—what works for you and yours. Cherish those values and stick to them.

The values that a country holds dear can easily be reflected by the way its children are nurtured. A report written by President Bill Clinton and posted on his website (clintonfoundation.org; click on "Fighting Childhood Obesity" on the home page) says Americans are raising the first generation that may not outlive their parents. I have not been able to find solid data to back up this alarming statement, made in the context of a discussion of obesity; even so, we can be certain we are raising a generation of children who are the least healthy in decades. What kinds of lives will our children have?

I can't tell you how many times parents in my office have complained that their children won't eat quality food. The problem is that they are more concerned about upsetting the child than about nourishing them. They allow the youngster to make the decisions about what he or she will eat.

I don't know about you, but when I was a kid if the decision had been up to me my diet would have consisted of Twinkies, Snow Balls, and Ho Hos. Fortunately, the choice was not mine. Every day before school my dad prepared two eggs and toast for me; thanks to my parents' early intervention I do know how I like my eggs—sunny-side up! A cereal box of Cocoa Krispies or Lucky Charms never graced our kitchen—I don't think we ever ate anything from a package. (Except of course our Saturday Sweet Sixteen donuts extravaganza! Just proof that my parents understood the importance of balance.)

I remember visiting a neighborhood friend, and her mother made salad with iceberg lettuce and French dressing. I went berserk—I'd never tasted orange dressing from a bottle. I ran home and told my mother all about the wonderful, sweet dressing and crispy lettuce and asked her to buy it the next time she went grocery shopping. She looked at me as if I were stark raving mad. Salad dressing from a bottle? Never.

In French restaurants children as young as five years of age place napkins on their laps, eat in courses, properly maneuver their utensils, and behave quite like the adults who accompany them. Chicken nuggets are nowhere to be found. Their young palates are much too sophisticated for kiddie food.

Le Déjuener à l'École: Lunch in a French School

Here is what I've learned from Jean Saunders, school wellness director for the Healthy Schools Campaign, about the way the French nurture and value their children. Jean attended the 2007 International Exchange Forum on Children, Obesity, Food Choice and the Environment in the Loire Valley of France.* This is the lunch she enjoyed at the junior high school, College Charles Milcendeau, in the municipality of Challans, on the western coast of France.

Salad of butter lettuce with smoked duck

Tomato and fresh mozzarella salad

Smoked salmon with asparagus and crème fraiche

Roasted chicken with roasted root vegetables and roasted potatoes

Apples with sabyon

Fresh strawberries

Goat cheese

French bread

Water

To paraphrase Jean's experience: A local farmer grows the butter lettuce, the strawberries are grown in the south of France, and the chicken (also grown locally)

is roasted whole. This wonderful meal is served on real plates accompanied by real cutlery and glassware. And the plates are warmed in a plate warmer. The kitchen has a veggie walk-in that holds *mâche*, a delicate and costly sweet, nutty salad green, and individual pantries and refrigeration for meat, dairy products, and other vegetables. Nothing is frozen or pre-made.

On July 2, 2008, Eleanor Beardsley, NPR's reporter of French culture and gastronomy, explained in a piece called "Chef Proves School Lunch Can Be Healthy" that this amazing French school food is prepared by French chefs—each school has one, and every two weeks the students are asked to weigh in on the food program. Chef Dominique Valadier, head chef at Lycée de Emperi, in the southern French provincial town of Salon de Provence, shops for fresh ingredients each morning. Valadier once worked in the glamorous world of Riviera restaurants. He says he left that life for something more meaningful. Investing in students' well-being is also an act of citizenship, he explains. If young people learn to eat well early on, they will cost the country's health care system a lot less in the future. Eleanor Beardsley lives in Paris with her husband and child and has been reporting from France since June 2004. She says that she can't think of a better place to raise a child than Paris.

Where the French girl seeks culture or knowledge, we [Americans] seek self-improvement, self-help. To unleash her, we don't have to act French, or (God forbid) pretend to be French. But we might want to rethink our values. Reject certain aspects of the status quo. Reposition ourselves against the currents (raging at times) that pull us away from our center. Edith Wharton reminds us that the four words that preponderate in French speech and literature are: glory, love, voluptuousness, and pleasure. Add to that self-possession, discretion, authenticity, and sensuality and you're well on your way to finding your inner French girl.
—Debra Ollivier, *Entre Nous*

Chef, writer, and teacher Deborah Madison reports that in addition to providing delicious food, school lunchrooms in France are brightly decorated, and the chairs are adjustable so that each child is comfortably positioned at the table.* Ceilings are fitted with acoustic tiles that reduce noise. All children, regardless of their parents'

income, are served meals that cost about three times what American school lunches do. The cost is shared among local government bodies, such as the mayor's office.

Two hours are dedicated to lunch and exercise. Teachers eat in their own rooms, but there is a core group of women—similar to our lunch moms—who are there just to be ready to lend a hand. They help smaller children with their food and answer questions; in the case of one boy who brought his lunch to school, the lunch mom reassigned it to a plate like the ones the other children had.

Through this whole approach to lunch—the exceptional food, the bright and inspirational setting, the caring lunch moms, and the excellent chefs—the French send a deep message of caring to their children.

Deborah said that, unfortunately, American children receive an entirely different message that is something more like, "We have to feed you something. It's gotta be cheap, and we don't really care about it or you."

On a good day in Osceola County, in central Florida, children can expect this menu:

Chili with grilled cheese sandwich
Mini corndogs
Garden salad
Coleslaw
Mixed fruit
Milk choice

I can assure you that the corndogs are not organic, nor is the fruit fresh. In nearby Orange County, the school system serves about 136,000 meals per day. The senior director of food and nutritional services, Lora Gilbert, is very proud of the fact that the students have a great deal of influence on their cafeteria's lunch menus. The suggestions of the students are tested in five or six schools, where a 70 percent acceptance rate is required. I guess that explains why they serve a lot of pizza.

As I said, if it had been up to me as a kid I'd be among the 70 percent voting for Ho Hos. Only thirty minutes are allowed for lunch in the U.S. public school system, and Ho Hos would certainly help the kids meet the efficiency standard.

In 2007, Orange County officials distributed water pouches as an FCAT (Florida Comprehensive Assessment Test) snack. Once the pouches were punched with straws they became water cannons. That snack idea was immediately scrapped. Where are the lunch moms when you need them?

The April 2010 issue of *Orlando Magazine* reported that Lora Gilbert visited an elementary school the first day corn on the cob was served there. "As I began explaining that corn came from a plant in the ground, one little girl immediately spit hers out, saying, 'I'm not eating something that came out of the dirt!'"

Respecting Your Food

Underlying the food culture in France is the belief that food and dining deserve respect. People express this respect by taking the time to eat and enjoy eating, apart from any other activity. Mealtime is an opportunity for children to relax, to enjoy, and simply to be. They are not distracted by anything other than themselves and a nurturing environment.

In France, school meals are *important*. The French spend more on school lunches than we do and use school meals as an educational tool to instill proper eating habits and good manners. French government recommendations acknowledge that students only eat one meal each day at school. The purpose of that meal, then, is to "assure an elementary formation of taste" and provide nutrition education. Lunches should incorporate lessons on the vocabulary of taste, regional specialties, food preparation techniques, and culinary heritage, the government suggests, adding that the midday meal "is much more than nutrients and calories."

That is in stark contrast to America's school lunch program, which is based on feeding students so they'll be able to focus in the classroom, rather than teaching them how to eat. Perhaps part of the emphasis on education in France comes from the strong culture and norms around eating. As Michael Pollan discusses in *In Defense of Food,* the United States doesn't have that kind of food tradition. We don't take pride in our cuisine, as the French do. Food just isn't very high on our list of priorities.

In February 2010, First Lady Michelle Obama recruited hundreds of chefs to join Let's Move, her anti-obesity campaign, part of which is an initiative to help schools serve healthier, tastier meals. Mrs. Obama has asked the chefs to partner with individual schools and to work with teachers and parents to help educate kids about food and nutrition; she made the point that healthy meals at schools are more important than ever today because many children get most of their calories there.

By February 2011, with a year under her belt, Mrs. Obama had some successes in her campaign against obesity, but more remained to be accomplished. In twelve months Obama moved the needle, with promises from food and beverage manufacturers, including Walmart, to reduce salt, fat, and sugar levels in products. The reality is that it takes time for lasting change. I do believe her message is getting through—we are, at the very least, in a conversation about how we make and sell food. Anti-obesity advocate Nancy Brown, CEO of the American Heart Association agrees, saying, "She has been a spark plug."*

AN AMERICAN IN PARIS: LESSONS LEARNED

"Off to the market the French go, choosing the specialties of the season, whether mushrooms or fruits and cheeses. They really plan it out, including the wine," my friend Susan said. "I started a habit of stopping by the wine shop to discuss what I was preparing for dinner guests; the proprietor always recommended wines for each course."

Susan shared a tip: "I learned to never offer a bottle of wine or champagne in your host's home as a gift. The hosts have carefully chosen every wine for each course to complement the meal. To bring wine is an insult. They feel they have to serve it, and it is awkward!"

"The French talk about the food, and every morsel is carefully seasoned and prepared. It never seemed complicated—simple but elegant," is how Susan described it. "We usually dined at about eight and relaxed at the table for hours. Time slips away, and the next thing you know, it is midnight," she said.

"What did you learn in France that you have kept as a practice in your current life?" I inquired.

Her reply: "To savor good wine and serve wine that complements what you have prepared."

Another great lesson: "It's hard to be heavy of heart when one is buoyed by the bubbles of champagne. And it should not be saved for special occasions. Every day should be celebrated, and one should always have a bottle or two chilling in the refrigerator—that's what I learned in France."

The celebrity chefs who joined Mrs. Obama picked arugula, baby spinach, rhubarb, and other vegetables from her garden on the White House lawn and showed the children how to wash, dice, and cook the veggies as together they made a grilled chicken salad and rhubarb crisp. Chef Todd Gray of the Washington restaurant Equinox spoke of his experience partnering with a local school. "It will change your life professionally and personally," he told the other chefs.

Progress Is on the Way

Congress gave final approval on December 2, 2010, to the Healthy, Hunger-Free Kids Act, a bill that reauthorizes the Child Nutrition Act, and President Obama signed it into law less than two weeks later. The bill will expand the school lunch program and set new standards to improve the quality of school meals, which will include more fruits and vegetables. It signifies a major move to revamp the future of school food. In a time when far too many children face both hunger and obesity, it presents an opportunity to set policy that will bring healthier food to the children who need it most.

What does this mean for schools? The reimbursements that schools receive for the meals they provide will increase by six cents per meal. Hopefully, we will see improved and sound nutrition standards for school meals. The legislation will enact policies that help schools send reliable messages about healthy eating throughout school buildings, including vending machines. It should help simplify the process by which children who are eligible for free meals get access to those meals. Plus, the bill includes pilot programs for expansion of farm-to-school programs as well as greater use of organic foods. As with most new initiatives, this is not a perfect bill, but it's a meaningful step in the right direction.

As a nutritionist and as a parent, I urge you to begin your child's love affair with food at home. After all is said and done, it is your responsibility to introduce your children to quality food and to develop an understanding that mealtimes are occasions for sharing, being nurtured, relaxing, and enjoying each other. Make certain that your children celebrate and appreciate what food producers—those who *grow food in the dirt*—have contributed to our tables, to our health, and to our lives.

Higher Knowledge

In April 2010, I watched Oprah interview Wes Moore, the author of *The Other Wes Moore*. The premise of Moore's book is that two young black men with the same name, coming up in the same area, ended up in very different places in life. One is serving a life sentence for his role in a jewelry store heist in which a guard was killed; the other, the author, ended up a Rhodes Scholar and White House Fellow. The book is a result of the author's desire to trace the histories and fates of the two men through an intriguing narrative designed to answer the question Moore asks himself, "What made the difference?"

Moore writes, "The truth is that I don't know." Oprah hints that education is the final answer, as if the years of Moore's reflection and investigation, not to mention the book itself, had not provided that rather obvious conclusion.

As I said, Moore is a Rhodes Scholar, so he didn't disagree with Oprah on national television about the fact that education played a part. "I think education taught me critical thinking. I think education showed me a world I never knew existed." Wes said. "My grandfather used to say that education is like a skeleton key. If you get that skeleton key it can open any door."

I, like Moore, agree that education is in fact the skeleton key to many successful outcomes, but I also reason that in our quest to educate ourselves, we neglect giving due credit to our values and wisdom. So often success is defined as what we know and have and, of course, how beautiful we are. We strive to possess the newest, shiniest, most technologically advanced objects, along with our prestigious diplomas. We tear down historic structures rather than embrace their character, just as we use plastic surgery to conceal our physical flaws. I believe that the roots of our ways of thinking lie in our value systems.

On May 19, 2010, U.S. Secretary of Education Arne Duncan announced that as many as 300,000 teachers could be laid off before the next school year began because states and cities do not have the money to pay for public education—this is the diet we are putting our children on. At the same time as we continue to fund two wars, bail out Wall Street, bail out the automakers, expand and privatize the state and federal prison systems, fund other countries' needs, including Israel's defense, at a cost of $3 billion a year, we increase classroom sizes and defend the poor-quality food we feed our children. Their minds and bodies are at stake. All we have to do is look at our actions; they speak volumes about our values.

I recently had a conversation with my husband in which he implied that Americans rally when there is a need—part of his effort to encourage me to believe there is hope for ending obesity in our children and for elevating the school lunch programs in this country. Yes, there are a few individuals, such as British celebrity chef Jamie Oliver, who are speaking out and sharing their concern. In the winter of 2009 Oliver turned his effort to transform the unhealthy diet of schoolchildren in a West Virginia town into a hit reality television program, *Jamie's Food Revolution*. Jamie traveled from the United Kingdom to America to raise awareness of the growing obesity crisis and aimed to get people cooking and eating good food again.

His mission was to start a chain reaction of positive change across the country. "The time is right for people to rediscover the sense of pride, satisfaction, and fun you can get from cooking for the people you love," he explains.

Jamie's philosophy is a bit like the French philosophy of eating. He believes that healthy eating has always been about enjoying everything in a balanced and sane way.

As he explains on his website jamieoliver.com: "Food is one of life's greatest joys, yet we've reached this really sad point where we're turning food into the enemy, and something to be afraid of. I believe that when you use good ingredients to make pasta dishes, salads, stews, burgers, grilled vegetables, fruit salads, and even outrageous cakes, they all have a place in our diets. We just need to rediscover our common sense: If you want to curl up and eat macaroni and cheese every once in a while—that's all right! Just have a sensible portion next to a fresh salad, and don't eat a big old helping of chocolate cake afterward."

Jamie inspires you to get in the kitchen and cook meals from scratch—no big deal. His demonstration of basic kitchen skills encourages the student or viewer to acquire a handful of favorite recipes in order to be able to prepare nutritious meals on any budget. His ultimate goal—"There's nothing like sitting around a table to bring people together," he says.

As of November 2011, nearly a million people around the world, including me, have signed his petition supporting the food revolution for better food at school and better health prospects.

Still, I wonder whether it is only after a catastrophe that we act. After the twin towers were destroyed we took the threats of terrorism seriously; after Katrina we thought about faulty levees. In both cases, the most educated of the educated had been in charge—the CIA, the FBI, the mostly highly trained, sophisticated, and educated structural engineers—supposedly taking actions that would have prevented these disasters. So it doesn't seem to be all about education.

When we turn that skeleton key and open the door to critical thinking, do we acknowledge our arrogance, greed, and our lack of values? I'm just asking. And then there's the most important question of all: Will we stand by and wait to rally until our children start to die?

Into the Onion

My research reminds me of an onion bulb. The more I peel the rounded bulb—first the dried and flaky brown skin, then the concentric layers beneath—the more the truth is exposed. The reality of my findings stings like the juice contained within the onion.

Do we really believe that the French Paradox unraveled is simply the presence of a few antioxidants or polyphenols in red wine? How can we possibly ignore that at the center of the obesity crisis is a crisis of values? It is, in fact, the entire *value* system of the French—the traditions, the rituals, and the respect for food, family, and life itself—that defines the country's achievement. No wonder we cry when peeling this onion back.

I know, I know, when you think about the French, philandering men and willing women come to mind, and what kind of a value is that, after all? Let's face it, French voters had no problem with the fact that Francois Mitterrand, who passed away in 1996 after having been France's longest-serving president, was married with children and also had a daughter with his mistress.

In our country we have seen the end of political careers too many to number as we uphold our steadfast pro-family values. In the United States a pro-family politician attends church regularly, opposes abortion, stem cell research, and gay marriage, and gives lip service to the sanctity of traditional marriage—and all the while he or she may be gay and/or adulterous.

As far as the French are concerned, these issues have little, if anything, to do with family values. For them, being pro-family means supporting policies that play a major role in helping parents and children in their daily lives—such as continued government support for universal medical care, state-run day care, family allowances to parents of young children to help them with the costs of raising children, social workers being available cost-free to help parents of newborns with child-rearing, free preschool programs for all children starting at age three, free education (elementary school through university, including graduate school, medical, law, and other professional schools), and a work year of approximately 1,440 hours and a minimum one month of paid vacation, which makes for more quality time for parents and children.

American "family values" conservatives would be quick to reject these kinds of benefits as constituting socialism and quick to point out France's enormous national debt and dysfunctional economy. A major part of France's national debt is caused by the services and benefits listed above, which are arguably investments in its future economic and social well-being, while a major part of our national debt is due to Pentagon spending.

A head-to-head comparison between the economies of the United States and France shows that the big difference is in priorities, not performance. According to the Organization for Economic Cooperation and Development, productivity in France, measured as gross domestic product per hour worked, is actually a bit higher than in the United States.

When Dani, our foreign exchange student from Germany, lived with us in Chicago she made so many trips to the Clinique counter I considered buying stock in the company. She loved American cosmetics, American fashion, and, more than anything, American parties. I believe her main interest in the foreign exchange program may have had a lot to do with attending the high school prom! Here are a few more things European and French women like about us.

Our eccentricity
The American virtue of tenacity
The goodwill and hospitality we offer people from other countries
American literature
American-made cosmetics like Clinique,
Mac, and Bobbi Brown
American fashion: Levi's, Calvin Klein,
the Gap, and many others
Pop music
Our country's big open spaces
Classic Hollywood cinema
Health food

Even so, France's gross domestic product per person is well below that of the United States, but that's because French workers spend more time with their families. Unemployment is an issue in France; many who would like to work cannot. Others retire early, and full-time French workers work shorter weeks and take more vacations than full-time American workers. The point is that to the extent that the French have less income than we do, it is mainly a matter of choice.

The typical French family, without question, has less disposable income than an American family. This translates to lower levels of personal consumption, smaller cars, smaller houses and apartments, less eating out. But there are positive trade-offs for this lower level of consumption: French schools are good across the country. Parents have no worries about getting their children into a good school district, not to mention the lack of worry about losing health insurance or being driven into bankruptcy by medical bills.

But most important, the members of the typical French family are compensated for their lower income by having much more time together. Fully employed French workers average about seven weeks of paid vacation a year. In America that figure is less than four.

In the end we are talking about two highly productive societies that have made different trade-offs between work and family time. And there's a lot to be said for the French choice.

Values will *always* determine where we expend our energy and efforts (actions). Actions will *always* determine our outcomes. If we don't like the outcomes we are getting, we should take a look at our values and determine whether they need adjusting.

> Value + action = outcome
>
> Convenience (value) + fast food (action) = obesity (outcome)
>
> Instant gratification (value) + latest fad diet (action) = another dieting failure (outcome)

As long as convenience or instant gratification is more valuable to us than thoughtfulness and devotion, our outcomes will not change. Not until we reach the root cause—our personal value systems—will our outcomes and lives improve.

Eating from the Gardens of Good and Evil

Fundamentalist religions dictate strict doctrines and tenets that do not honor individualism and the human condition, making it impossible for some of their followers to endure as such for long. Think about the hypocrisy exhibited in the lives of Ted Haggard, Jimmy Swaggart, and Jim Bakker. The charge of hypocrisy leveled at some leaders of the church has become so pervasive that even Christian apologists feel obligated to address it.

In the same way, as a nutritionist I feel obligated to address the overly strict setting of standards for food—it's almost really a moralization of food—along with strict dictates and the holding up of impossible levels of compliance. As put forward by my industry, such standards and dictates take on an absolutism that can confer an almost supernatural quality on, say, a fad diet.

I am certainly not suggesting that Christianity's claims about the existence of God are false. The hypocrites within Christianity do, however, undermine a different supernatural claim: the alleged ability of Christian belief to transform *all* people's lives in a uniquely effective and beneficial way.

Neither am I saying that different foods do not have either positive or negative effects on health. What I am saying is that no food is morally good or morally corrupt. In the words of nutritional psychologist Marc David, "When people say sugar is bad, there is often a hidden judgment that sugar is evil. Sugar may have negative effects on health, but I know of no candy bars that ever conspired to rot people's teeth."

One more thought on the moralization of food: Buddha ate meat when it was offered to him, and Hitler was a vegetarian. So much for the stereotypes that define "kind" vegetarians and "cruel" meat eaters.

Life's meaning cannot be transferred to food—even the highest-quality food. Diets live outside of us, while nutrition and nurturance are an inside job. In dieting we check our power and sense of self at the door as we seek an easy way out—following a program built on another's concept of sustenance. Diets move in like cheap-shot artists who sidetrack our thoughts, our awareness, our love, our attention, and our spirit by providing an outside distraction. We focus on what goes into our stomach when it's our hearts that are crying for attention.

The point is that the second we label a food bad, we begin to fear it, think about it, fight it—and often crave it. We even go so far as to label anyone who eats this food a bad person. We set up an internal dynamic that in avoiding the food we are protecting ourselves. Most of our craving at this point is due to the fear of the food rather than the food itself. When we drop our fear and the belief that the food is evil, the desire is typically reduced and, in most cases, eliminated.

"Whenever we avoid anything," Marc David explains in his book *Nourishing Wisdom*, "a homeostatic mechanism is set off driving us to reunite with it. This is a deeply programmed feature of the mind that cannot be averted. For example, if someone we love insults us and we feel hate inside, it would seem as if hating them would barricade us from our thoughts. Yet the hate only makes us think of them more, and though they may have only insulted us once, we replay it over and over in our mind, in effect repeating the original offense perhaps hundreds of times. Our thoughts will focus on that person until it is integrated, resolved, and made neutral. The same with food."

I have shocked many a client by encouraging them to embrace and partake of a forbidden food with no restrictions. "My hunger is bottomless," they worry. "If I start eating I'll never stop."

"But how do you know that?" I counter. "Have you ever fully given in to your desire?"

For those who are willing to permit themselves to binge on their forbidden foods and enjoy them, the craving smothers itself. The pleasure simply wears off. The next time they eat the illicit food, the craving is radically diminished; it's easier to experience satisfaction and let go of anxieties.

As for me, I tackled one food at a time until my angst lifted. Before I knew it, the foods I feared remained in the pantry for weeks, maybe months. If I did decide to indulge, I was satisfied with a modest portion. I drowned out the messages from the media and well-meaning friends. I continued to eat consciously rather than critically.

Another important reason to address the moralization of food is that when we view a particular food as bad, we also view ourselves as bad for having the desire. The yo-yo dieting cycle is once again in motion—guilt, punishment, deprivation, and weight gain.

All America's Children

In the past ten years, an alarming number of adolescents and children have been diagnosed with eating disorders. A study reported in the journal of the American Academy of Pediatrics estimates that 0.5 percent of adolescent girls in the United States have anorexia nervosa, and 1 percent to 2 percent meet the criteria for bulimia nervosa.*

Perhaps even more shocking news from the same source: There is a growing awareness of eating disorders in males, who now account for 10 percent of all cases of eating disorders.

A recent examination by the Agency for Healthcare Research and Quality discovered that from 1999 to 2006, hospitalizations for eating disorders in children under twelve years of age increased by 119 percent. Consequently, our young children suffer with organ damage, stunted growth, and malnutrition. In some cases involving bulimia, a rapid change in electrolyte balance can cause heart attacks and sudden death. In 2005 and 2006 alone, 24 percent of eating disorder patients had cardiac dysrhythmias, an increase of 125 percent from 1999 and 2000. Also, 4 percent had acute renal or liver failure, an increase of 118 percent.*

If you think that your own preoccupation with diets and appearance has not contributed to the problem, I urge you to think again. Children learn most everything from their parents. The little they don't learn from you, they pick up from the media or their friends who have been influenced ahead of them. These prevailing influences, combined with the pressures of youth, serve as the perfect Petri dish in which obesity and eating disorders grow, thrive, and ultimately kill.

Revisit your values. Lift your children off the scales of judgment and into the safe haven of acceptance. Teach by example. Be a role model and a mentor for all of the young people you encounter and affect. Help prevent obesity and eating disorders in America by fostering only healthy eating attitudes.

Let go of the harsh scrutiny and unhealthy obsessions you inflict on yourself, for these are handed down to your young ones. Instead, as you develop your own interests, talents, and self-esteem, encourage your children to value their unique gifts.

There is no time like the present to make a difference in the lives of our children while creating a lasting footprint for future generations.

PRACTICING YOUR FRENCH

This week:

1. Take the time to identify and document your core values. Apply this equation: value + action = outcome.
2. Determine how your current core values may be affecting your weight-management efforts as well as your life as a whole.

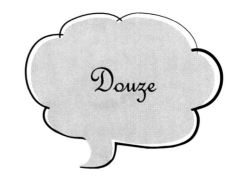

Manger à la Française
Eating the French Way

*To invite a person into your home
is to take charge of his happiness for
as long as he is under your roof.*
—Jean Anthelme Brillat-Savarin

THE FINAL SECRET in my book is a simple summary of all that has come before: Eat the French way.

When the French eat at home, they pride themselves on making mealtime a memorable and positive experience. For everyday lunches and dinners, four courses are typically served: salad, a main dish with meat, cheese with bread, and a dessert. Bread and water are always served. Special occasions include even more courses, such as an appetizer of savory pastries or other finger foods. Meals are normally served with an alcoholic beverage, often a French wine. Several bottles of wine may be served with the meal. Coffee is also served.

In French restaurants, it is expected that patrons are there to enjoy a full meal. Diners typically order wine by the half or full bottle or carafe (a glass container that comes in various sizes and that is designed to allow the wine to "breathe"). They rarely tip waiters; restaurants in France generally add a fee for service to the bill.

Eating out is a social occasion and, while restaurants in France are generally more formal than those in the United States, is a leisurely activity. It is considered rude to ask to have leftover food wrapped to be taken home.

JE SAIS CUISINER

Ginette Mathiot's *Je Sais Cuisiner* has been the cooking bible for three generations of French families. First published in 1932, it continues to be a must for anyone setting up a new home and is an essential fixture on the counters of French kitchens. Now the first English edition, published in 2009 as *I Know How to Cook*, reveals for English-speaking readers the secrets of simple, delicious French home cooking, from *croquet monsieur* to *cassoulet*.

Les Repas Quotidien: Daily Meals in France

The typical eating habits of the French include three meals a day, plus *le goûter*.

Le Petit Déjeuner: *Breakfast*

The typical French breakfast, which features fresh bread, is a simple one eaten *en famille*. The French prefer a light, white, crusty bread that tends to go stale in only a few hours. The classic way to deal with this problem is to make the loaves thicker. By managing the ratio of crust to crumb in favor of crumb—making the interior volume proportionally greater than the surface area—the bread near the surface may start to go stale but the interior is preserved.

It follows that people who live a long way from a bakery and might shop for bread once a week prefer loaves that are up to a foot thick. Parisians, on the other hand, who are seldom more than 200 yards from a bakery, can buy fresh bread for each meal and choose very thin, crispy loaves.

The bread most desired for breakfast is the baguette, a loaf about two feet long and two to three inches wide. For breakfast it is cut into *tartines*, segments six inches long that are split down the middle and spread with real butter and homemade fruit preserves.

A classic French breakfast may also include croissants or pains au chocolat or pains au raisin, again with jam. Croissants are not to be buttered, because they are already one-third butter, and to add more would be absurd, even for the French. Fresh fruit and yogurt are also commonly served. A large breakfast is rare, and eggs are eaten more often in the evening than the morning.

Before you get too excited, let me tell you what Requia Badr noted: "I remember the first time I traveled to Los Angeles. We had a breakfast in a restaurant on Sunset Boulevard and a friend ordered for us a French pastry (just to taste the French pastries prepared by an American chef), an almond croissant. I was really amazed by the size of the croissant and I was unable to finish it! I think in France, the same piece will be called a *giant* almond croissant."

As a breakfast beverage, tea is common and hot chocolate even more so, especially for children. But the standard drink is coffee, *café*, usually very strong; *café au lait* is coffee served with hot milk, generally in a bowl-size cup. French coffee during the rest of the day is inclined to be strong and enjoyed in small quantities.

Le Déjeuner: *Lunch*

The main meal of the day in France, lunch takes more time to eat than the typical lunch in the United States. For this reason, many businesses close between 12 noon and 2 P.M. A leisurely affair, lunch includes several courses. The first, called the *hors d'oeuvre*, is often a salad; in winter, it might be a bowl of soup. A main dish of meat or fish follows, and the meal ends with a triangle of creamy cheese and a square of dark chocolate, fruit, or sometimes a more complicated dessert.

Le Goûter: *The Snack (the Equivalent of English Teatime)*

Between 3:30 P.M. and 4:00 P.M. every day, when the typical American is eating a candy bar, the French are in a café sipping on tea, espresso, or hot chocolate and maybe eating a *macaron*. Children who have just returned from school might have some bread with jam or chocolate, and a glass of milk. This is a time to rest, regroup, socialize, or just enjoy one's own company. It is as much about ritual as it is about substance. *Le goûter* is delicious enough to hold one over until dinner but not large enough to spoil the appetite.

The French tend to snack much less than Americans; instead, they try to eat more regularly. If they do snack, they often have a piece of fresh fruit.

Le Dîner: *Dinner*

For many French people, the evening meal is a time for the whole family to gather and talk about their day. Depending on how big lunch was, dinner may consist of several courses and, for the adults, might be accompanied by a glass or two of wine.

Setting aside half an hour or so before a meal for *l'apéritif* is a national custom in France. People cherish these moments when they share a drink, a few bites, and conversation with family, friends, neighbors, or colleagues. Kir (white wine with cassis) is popular in Paris, whereas in the South of France pastis (made with anise) is the official aperitif. Other popular aperitifs are whiskey, martinis, and port wine. Champagne is served for special events as an aperitif or with dessert. This firmly established social activity is enjoyed by people of all ages and forms an important part of home life, of public and private celebrations, and of café and restaurant culture.

There are no kid-friendly menus in France and, even more astonishing, no whining or tantrums. Children sit down politely and, if old enough to read, order from the same menu as their parents. The younger children are fed directly from their parents' plates. Children enjoy the same food as adults—salads, fresh fish, roasted chicken, quiche, and fresh vegetables, eaten in courses.

The French drink a lot of bottled water rather than sodas; they consume on average 52 liters of soft drinks per person annually, compared with 216 liters per person in the United States. On the other hand, the intake of bottled water is very high in France (147 liters per person annually) and low in the U.S. (46.8 liters per person).

Off to Market

Somehow we have been given an image of the typical French cook, wicker basket in tow, lingering in an open-air market every morning, buying everything freshly harvested and sharing recipes with the farmers. Well, maybe at one time that was the case. But today's French woman is no different than her American counterpart. She has a career, a family, and many diverse interests. So how does she find the time to shop?

Clotilde Dusoulier says, "I think this is mostly a myth, based on a truth from a long, long, time ago. What a lot of French people do nowadays is diversify their sources for food. They will buy most things at the grocery store, some from local shops or at the market (bread, meat, fish, produce, cheese, wine), and some from local producers even (if they live in a region where there are any). But since most of these things are available from the grocery store (and some supermarkets have a very good selection of fresh products), many people do all of their shopping there because it's more convenient."

She continues, "I do some of my shopping at the grocery store, but I try to support my local food shops by buying from them what they are specialized in. For instance, I would rather buy cheese from the *fromagerie*, meat from the *boucherie*, and produce from the open-air market than buy them at the grocery store. It is more time-consuming (several stops versus just one) and usually more expensive (though not always), but the products are better quality, and I enjoy the advice and human contact."

"When I was living with my parents," Estelle Tracy begins, "we used to go shopping every Saturday. In the morning we would go to the *marché* (open-air market where local producers sell their fruits and vegetables) to buy some produce. Then, we would go to the grocery store to buy our pantry items, plus some fruits and vegetables, as they would be sometimes cheaper than at the *marché*. Overall, I think that most French people do not go to the markets every day—unless they are retired and are lucky enough to have such markets open every day. Even though French people are, in my opinion, pickier than the Americans about their food, they don't have much more time to devote to their shopping.

"It is, however, true that open-air markets are popular in France, and it is customary for people to buy their produce there. The food is usually fresher and the contact with the sellers friendlier than at the grocery store. But since the grocery stores are usually cheaper than *marchés*, lots of people actually buy their produce or their meat in supermarkets." Commenting on her American experience, Estelle goes on to say, "In the U.S., *marchés* don't exist, and butcher shops and bakeries are not common either, so the only option is really to go to the grocery store. I have been in various farmers' markets several times, but the quality was disappointing and the prices were a little too high for me."

Referring to her American workplace, Estelle explains, "There is no cafeteria, and I am lucky enough to work almost across from a Whole Foods market. I usually have lunch there and shop a little every day. I think that produce is really expensive in American grocery stores, but fortunately I found some local produce markets that are much cheaper than the grocery stores. That's the only way for me to eat healthy and cheap. I am still searching for a good baguette, though."

Requia Badr says, "I buy fresh products as often as I can. Every Sunday morning we used to go to market and buy fresh fruits and fresh vegetables for the next week and meat for the following days. I never buy meat or bread in the supermarket, but only at the butcher and bakery. I took this habit from my mum; when I was younger, the market was a fun time I would spend with my mum. What's more, my father is, let's say, a gardening addict, so we always ate fresh fruits and vegetables at home, and I try to keep this good habit today in my home with my husband."

"Of course, I can only answer for myself," Pascale Weeks establishes. "It's true that we have a lot of markets here in France. Each town—even small towns—have their own market at least twice a week. When I was working I used to go to the market every weekend, either on a Saturday or Sunday morning. Now I go to the market twice a week. I buy all the vegetables and fruits, all the fish, half the meat and cheese. I buy all the rest in supermarkets, except bread, which I buy in a bakery, or wine, which I buy at the local wine store. Markets are very famous in France, as you find a wider variety of fruits or vegetable and at a better quality. It's also a place where you can ask a lot of questions about how to cook the products and where they come from. On the other hand, I know some people who buy all their food in supermarkets because they find it easier to buy everything at the same place. It's a question of choice, but at least we have the choice."

What I have learned from Estelle, Clotilde, Pascale, and Requia is that they value not only the quality of the fresh, whole ingredients they gather, but also the joy associated with shopping and selecting the food that will nourish their families. As Requia describes the fun she enjoyed with her mother while shopping, the rhythms and rituals of the French surface again. Perhaps we can find the same sort of joy in our shopping experience by creating a new family ritual that becomes less a chore and more a thoughtful part of a meaningful relationship with food.

La Manière Française: The French Way

"Where's the plan?" you ask, flipping frantically through the pages. There must be a chapter that divulges the secret steps, maybe a workshop or, better yet, a prescription of cabbage soup promising detoxification in a mere seven days. Just enough to kick-start weight loss.

First, stop, drop, and roll down memory lane until you're back to when you last started a diet. It's Monday, and you enthusiastically approach the new plan, encouraged because the people in the television ad lost so much weight quickly. This is "the one."

By Wednesday it's another story altogether—this is a lot harder than you'd expected. And you're hungry. But you persevere in a self-righteous sort of way, ignoring your growling belly. Riding it out is a sort of high in and of itself.

A few days later, things are looking up, or rather down, on the scale, and for a fleeting moment you are feeling just a little superior to the rest of us.

Not so fast, you learn. Out of the blue—corn chips, from seemingly nowhere. Just when you were on top of the world, you caved and devoured the entire bag.

"I am a loser, a failure, an unfortunate creature born without willpower," you concede, sobbing while suffering from a stomachache and salty, cracked lips.

"See, I was better off on the diet," you presume. "I've learned my lesson. I'll be better next time. Tomorrow I'll do it right."

Once again you're caught up in the allure of a fresh start, a clean slate, a near-empty plate. Tomorrow is the day. And so goes the endless loop of victimization, concession, a new diet, and false pride, along with the fleeting high of rejecting food. Tomorrow. Always tomorrow.

Dieting is a bad idea, and unfortunately nothing dies harder than a bad idea.

Instant gratification, false promises, quick fixes, celebrity endorsements, and someone else's program—including mine—will never, ever define success or sustainability for *you*. Look at it this way, when I go to the gym and work out, I build the muscle and I benefit from the workout. In order for *you* to build the mental muscle, integrate the core principles, and achieve a successful outcome, *you* must perform the scrutinizing, the assessment, and the heavy lifting.

In writing this book, I chose the French food culture as my reference for two main reasons. First and most important, I have found through my personal experience in traveling to France and in subsequently practicing effortless weight management that this approach resonates with *me*. Second, I appreciate and respect the fact that science validates the gastronomical practices of a society immersed in centuries of extraordinary culinary tradition.

There may be an equally valid health-supportive program that resonates with you; if so, let that be your launching pad while allowing the fundamentals of this book to supplement your alternative program. The Mediterranean and Okinawan cultures also have evolved diets that result in health and longevity; neither promotes deprivation, and each is focused on real, high-quality, non-processed food enjoyed in modest portions. I just like the idea of a French pastry *ménage a trois* now and again!

Another important criterion is remaining true to the ultimate goal—staying clear of any plan or culture resembling anything close to restrictive eating. This includes any strategy that eliminates an entire food group or requires weighing yourself or your food, counting calories, carb grams, fat grams, or points, or a devotion to the glycemic index.

The French way of eating is based on values that include variety, pleasure, freedom, individualism, health, family, relaxation, socialization, and indulgence.

What Will Your Plan Be?

In order to lighten up, lighten up.
—Alan Cohen

It goes without saying that foremost in establishing your eating intention is the need to, first, define your unique personal value system. That solid foundation will support your life as a whole as well as your nutritional goals. If your house is not designed and built upon a well-considered personal value system, it will likely be constructed on shifting sand; it's likely to be here today and gone tomorrow.

Consider some of the following values, taking note of the ideals of the French (on the left) compared to those associated with restrictive dieting (on the right).

Self-discipline	Impulsivity
Patience	Instant gratification
Self-possession	Insecurity
Authenticity	Imitation
Quality	Quantity
Moderation	Greed
Freedom	Imprisonment
Choice	Willpower
Mindfulness	Absence
Balance	Instability
Discipline	Chaos
Real	Processed
Peace	Drama
Judgment	Acceptance

As you contemplate the right eating plan for you, devote time on the front end to an honest assessment of your behavior. Your choices and your values have consequences, so select carefully. The evidence of misplaced values surrounds us. Consider the state of obesity in America today—what are the values our country holds dear? As a nation, what values do we truly honor? If you value limitation, for example, restrictive diets will appeal to you. If freedom and flexibility sound more like it, read on!

AN AMERICAN IN PARIS: A FRENCH CHRISTMAS

"The first year it was Notre Dame Cathedral, and we walked home along the Seine in the wee hours of the morning. The markets were aglow with holiday lights stretching across the streets like banners," Susan remembered.

"One year we went to a small Italian church, and it was beautiful. The priest prepared the sacraments while singing Christian holiday songs," she reflected. "To hear him sing *Silent Night* in Italian was so emotional for me. The others sang the same chorus in French simultaneously—the sound was that of angels. Of course, I had to chime in, singing it in English in my tiny voice from the back of the church. Afterward cookies were served downstairs. I can honestly say that, despite being so far away from my family, I was never closer to the Christmas spirit."

The single most important determining factor in your life is you, and you are not a victim. Know who you really are. Know what you can and cannot live with.

After years of discounting your power you may be filled with self-doubt and fear. There is nothing better for building self-worth, courage, and empowerment than bestowing on yourself the gift of time and attention and thus investing in your own life and character. The simple, positive, everyday actions that result from this process, taken one step at a time, will result in a meaningful life, one that is rich, happy, whole, and diet free.

A winning plan approaches food as your ally, teacher, and rudder. It will nourish you when well chosen; if incorrectly chosen, it will teach you lessons that you may or may not heed. If you make a mistake in your food selection, either perversely or in ignorance, you will have to pay with an aching stomach or excess pounds, so why feel guilty on top of that? The results of your eating choices, if negative, should be considered information, not punishment.

Replace criticism of yourself with curiosity about food and how your body enjoys and uses it.

Effortless weight management is a simple and *natural* process. Animals rely on their instincts in maintaining their dietary needs; if we take the time to learn this technique from them they may have taught us more than the "diet experts" ever can. Unfortunately, the American culture supports and businesses profit from an astounding number of confusing, convoluted, elaborate, and expensive diet programs, and tons of exercise paraphernalia—useless distractions from the real work that people must do to gain control of their bodies.

The truth is, a proper and successful plan is easily executed quietly, simply, individually, and without fanfare. It's the way the French have eaten for centuries.

Eating Is Like Making Love

When my husband had started working at his new office in Manhattan but I hadn't yet left our place in Florida, I flew up to join him for a couple of days in the city; the goal was to grab a break from my work on the book—just get away, really. With Kindle in hand, I boarded the plane for LaGuardia and considered my reading options. I settled on *All You Need to Be Impossibly French: A Witty Investigation into the Lives, Lusts, and Little Secrets of French Women*, by Helena Frith-Powell. Okay, it's not exactly getting away from my book research, but the funny and entertaining, albeit stereotypical accounting of the secret lives of French women kept my attention on the much-too-early morning flight, and that's what mattered most. I highlighted a few paragraphs on the necessity of silk undies as well as the miracle of face and body creams, relieved that the shops of Madison, Park, and Fifth were just a few hours away. It was time to tweak my outer French girl.

With due respect to my French experiment, I headed off in a fashionably chic pair of flats and carrying a great handbag, ready for a day of shopping, primping, and dining—of course! I kissed my husband good-bye in front of his office building and continued uptown to Blow for a do at the blow-dry bar—of course! I have to tell you, this is one of the very best concepts I have ever encountered. Just pop in, drop your head in a shampoo bowl, and get the shampoo and style of your life. Bonnie, my hairdresser, shampooed my hair *twice*, then tugged and twirled my thick tresses for about thirty minutes. I bounced out with the locks of a fashion model. *Par excellence!*

Serious about validating my French philosophy, I hoofed it for the entire day. My iPhone indicated the walk from my husband's office to Blow to be 3.5 miles, and my rough calculations meant I would log at least 8 miles for the day. The thought alone sent me straight to a bistro. I grabbed a cold Perrier and a baguette filled with cheese, tomato, and olive, saving dessert for later in the day. I continued uptown to Clyde's, my favorite *pharmacie*, for a look at the latest potions and then worked my way through midtown, weaving in and out of shops along the way. "How do French women do this each and every day in heels," I wondered. My feet were screaming in my cute flats.

The melody of the dinging department store bells in Saks Fifth Avenue took my mind away from my throbbing feet and legs long enough for me to arrive at the lingerie department. As I summed up the offerings, my attention wandered in gratitude to Madame Herminie Cadolle, a French woman (naturally), who in 1889, is said to have pulled us out of the corset and into the bra, which in my opinion remains a medieval contraption. Nevertheless, I was there to embrace intimate apparel as the foundation of a proper and seductive French wardrobe. With the assistance of a very knowledgeable sales staff, I chose a cute ensemble that fits well and highlights the good stuff.

"Should I send a note to the executives at Saks?" I wondered. The lighting in the dressing rooms is horrid. In her book Helena Frith-Powell tells us that in the Galeries LaFayette in Paris, the changing rooms have two buttons on the wall; one summons an assistant, and the other changes the light inside the cubicle from day to night so you can see at the flick of a switch how you will look when your lover undresses you. These French people are the most *brilliant* people who have graced the earth, I decide.

My inner timepiece urged me to stop for *le goûter*, and as luck would have it there is a lovely chocolate bar on the fifth floor of Saks, right outside the shoe department. The only shoes that I might have been interested in at that moment were house slippers, so I bypassed the shoe selection, maybe for the first time in my entire life, and took a seat at the counter. As plated desserts covered in shiny glass domes made their way in front of and around me on a conveyor belt, I ordered a cappuccino with real sugar, quite proud to be off the artificial stuff.

The selections circled: two beautifully plated chocolate brownie triangles, a white chocolate and cranberry scone, a cinnamon-sugar French muffin, and a rather large American-style cookie. I took a picture with my iPhone to send my cousin Trish, hoping to make her jealous, and shot off a quick "look at this" email. Finally I choose—what else?—the *French* muffin, a luscious choice and perfect accompaniment to the cappuccino. I think I'm getting the hang of this French stuff.

I departed with my taste buds and ego satisfied. "You look so familiar, like a famous person—who are you?" the giddy young lady who served me asked.

Eating is like making love. In France
we put our whole bodies and minds into
experiencing good food and wine. The French
don't eat just to fill their bellies or because
it's time but to enjoy the experience. We
savor both the food and the experience.

—Chef Alain Sailhac,
Provost and Senior Dean of Culinary Studies,
French Culinary Institute

"Not famous," I replied, "but let's pretend I am." I laughed as I thought about what a good blow-dry does for a girl. She eagerly jumped on the suggestion, throwing out possibilities as I waved *au revoir*.

My purchases of the day consisted of a b. tempt'd by Wacoal lacy black and pink bra and matching panties, two Laura Mercier lip liners, and a Longchamp tote. As I unpacked my bags I remembered peering into the window of an Italian café, longing for the fresh pasta dish the couple shared.

I phoned my husband, telling him that I was home from my excursion and that my taste buds were crying for some fresh pasta; I suspected he was in the mood for sushi. With a few minutes to spare before he arrived, I slipped into the bath, soaking my feet and dreading the thought of putting my shoes back on for the evening. So instead, I tried on my new lingerie just in time for my husband's homecoming. Suffice it to say, he b. tempt'd!

Following the perfectly coiffed bouncy hair, lacy lingerie liaison I could have suggested dog doo doo for dinner and it would have been great by my husband. "These French women *are* brilliant," I determined once and for all. Still, I needed a break from my French obsession, so I stuck with my craving, something closer to my heritage—Italian, and specifically pasta.

Casa Lever would be just the thing to indulge my Italian fix. Sam Sifton, the restaurant critic for the *New York Times* named Casa Lever one of his "Sifty Fifty" favorites in New York City, so why not? "OK, let's go!" my husband agreed, with a silly grin plastered on his face. "Ya wanna walk?"

My response was something like, "Are you kidding? My feet are stubs!" After promising me a foot massage, my husband grabbed some cash from the ATM, handed me some bills for tomorrow's shopping (read more lingerie), and we hailed a cab to Lever House on Park Avenue.

An Italian host escorted us to a small table along a long wall, where, upon sitting, I immediately and covertly slipped off my high heels. Using my interest in the Andy Warhol prints, I admired the artwork that decorated the cavernous yet cozy room while I searched the plates of the diners already served for inspiration.

Our engaging waiter shared the specials, the first a salad with roasted quail and fig that sounded great to me, minus the quail. There were few salad selections on the menu, so I decided that if we shared the salad, my husband would eat the majority of the little bird. We ordered the quail salad special, and I choose a pasta dish. My husband ordered the veal Milanese, and we relaxed, forgoing wine for a large bottle of sparkling water as our beverage.

Not long after our quail salad arrived—and I must say it was beautiful and tasty—a couple was seated next to us. The tiny space between the tables meant that this was a bit of a squeeze; the pair had a brief word and the gentleman insisted the lady have the view of the room. No problem there; she was the size of Olive Oyl and slipped gracefully into the bench seat like a limbo champ. As intimate as the seating arrangement was, I don't believe either one ever looked our way or beyond the confines of their small table. Still, the position of the tables allowed us to hear every word they said—every *French* word, that is.

I couldn't stop myself—the two became immediate subjects for a case study, beginning with the gentleman's request for a salad of something simple, while the lady ordered the soup du jour. The congenial waiter was more than happy to oblige, and when the gentleman was presented with a lovely frisée salad I asked myself why I didn't request a salad to my liking.

The discussion the pair engaged in was so captivating that when they were served it took minutes—I mean like seven or eight—for either one of them to begin eating their starter. I was anxious, fearing the soup would be cold before she ever tasted it. Finally, the gentleman picked up his fork and took a bite of the salad. The lady continued talking, leaning over the table toward her partner, her willowy arms stretching as she clasped and wrung her hands expressively. His eyes never left hers, and I realized that although he was as short as Popeye and no better-looking, his interest in her every word transformed him into a most attractive man. As I observed the two of them I imagined Olive Oyl in some red satin lingerie under her prim and proper simple black dress. Madame Oyl savored about three tablespoons of soup before offering it to Monsieur Sailor Man, who was happy to oblige. Gee, I wonder why French women don't get fat!

Soon after, the discussion revolved around the wine selection, with the diners clearly questioning the server's recommendation. Out of his league and catching on quickly, the waiter offered each a taste of his suggestion. As he scurried away the expressions of the two were serious and somber, as if they had just heard some very bad news. The waiter returned with two wine goblets and a splash of red wine. The lady took the first sip as the gentlemen swirled and sniffed. The sour look on the gentleman's face matched his conclusion. "It's tart," he stated politely, as the waiter fumbled, retrieving the glasses. The lady remained serious, perplexed and now just a little more assertive in her preferences for what was clearly intended as the *pièce de résistance* of their dining experience. The three agreed on a different selection, and another round of tasting.

In the meantime, a beautiful plate of symmetrically sliced tomatoes was presented; a drizzle of olive oil with some freshly ground sea salt and pepper added the finishing touch. "I don't remember seeing that on the menu," I whispered to John.

"That's because it wasn't on the menu," he answered. The couple knew exactly what they wanted—just excellent ingredients served plain on a plate. They selected and substituted without self-consciousness or apologies, as if their lives depended on it.

The next wine option was presented, and the two accepted it. Though it's my guess that it was not up to their usual standard, they were polite and seemed to accept the "good enough" wine.

We observed their entrée selection; the lady chose the fish special—a 4-ounce portion served on a bed of vegetables—while her partner had a modest portion of pasta. Again, the conversation trumped the food, and a few minutes passed until they began eating. By this time our check had arrived. My eyes were sore from my pigeon stare, and though disappointed that I couldn't observe my subjects' dessert ritual, I resigned myself with the justification that this evening was intended to be a night off, after all. Believe it or not, my husband convinced me into walking the mile or so home where we chatted about Popeye and Olive Oyl all the way.

"He was so engaged," I said of the gentleman. "Forget his looks. If I were single, I would date him for that alone," I confided in my husband. Fortunately, my husband was still basking in the glow of our earlier rendezvous, and his ego was intact. As he laughed and I limped back to the hotel, he responded with a confident chuckle, "Well, you're not single, and although you're practically French, you're on your way home with me!"

PRACTICING YOUR FRENCH

This week:

1. Find a local farmers' market and become a regular. Let your senses do the shopping by building a meal around the freshest food of the season.
2. Buy something typically French you've never eaten and cook with it. Start by sprinkling some herbes de Provence on your chicken or egg dishes.
3. Invest in a beautiful French basket or shopping tote. For a wide variety of beautiful handmade market baskets, check out jeannebeatrice.com. These baskets are light, sturdy, eco-friendly, very French, and a great way to kick off a new market ritual.

Wishing You Freedom, Passion, and Life in Body and Soul

I DASHED OUT OF the duty-free shop at the Charles de Gaulle airport clutching my last little memento of Paris—a bottle of Hermes Caléche parfum. John relaxed nearby at a small table with the newspaper and espresso. I joined him, flaunting my prize, as we enjoyed our last hour in Paris, in the library-quiet airport.

"Something feels strange," John noted.

I said, "Yeah, I can't put my finger on it. It's very serene and calm here, isn't it?" We picked up our newspapers and continued reading.

"But it's an airport," my husband continued. "And yet I haven't heard one flight called over the loudspeaker."

And he was correct, because there were no loudspeakers. Only a discreet information board where it is up to each traveler to consult the display for flight updates. No screeching microphones calling out orders—just order alone. No following the crowd, but instead finding one's own way.

Since that day in Paris, I began to find my way. "Eating the French way" meant leaving my baggage behind. I have slowed down; I have turned off the loudspeakers and allowed my intuition to take precedence over my logical mind.

I have accepted that lifelong effortless weight management is to a large degree an informed, committed decision. Serenely, respectfully, comfortably, and individually I have embraced a culture of self-defined values. I have adopted the *value* of good health and all that accompanies it.

Just as I found my course in Paris, I wish you the very best in finding your way to a comfortable, health-supportive relationship with food. Leave the crowd in the dust, say no to restrictive dieting, no to deprivation drama and carbohydrate chaos. Taste and savor freedom, passion, and life in body and soul. ✄

Appendix
Body and Beauty Foods

Hᴇʀᴇ's ᴀ sᴛʀᴇᴀᴍʟɪɴᴇᴅ rundown of foods with decided benefits, noted as their key nutritional elements. Including them in your diet will improve your health and enhance your appearance. (Add high-fiber foods to your eating plan gradually, in order to allow your digestive system to naturally adapt to the benefits of increased roughage in the colon.)

Apples

- Protect the heart. Recommended for anyone with high blood cholesterol or blood-glucose problems such as hypoglycemia or diabetes. For weight watchers, good to eat just before meals, as they blunt the appetite, and as a between-meal snack.
- Fiber: a medium apple provides 15 percent of the daily recommendation; some of this is soluble fiber, which may help lower blood cholesterol.
- Pectin: rich in this soluble fiber. Eating two apples a day pushes enough pectin through the blood to make a real dent in cholesterol levels for some people.
- Rich in vitamin C, plus worthwhile amounts of vitamin E.

Apricots

- ❧ Provide flavonoids, which strengthen capillaries, reducing the risk of bruising and bleeding.
- ❧ Beta-carotene: good for the eyes, bones, and teeth and for boosting immune function.
- ❧ Vitamin C: used in the manufacture of collagen, the "glue" that gives skin its elasticity and support; vital for wound healing and protection against infection.

Bananas

- ❧ Pectin: a higher pectin content even than apples. Sweet, filling, sustaining, and easy to digest, a good food for anyone who suffers from acid indigestion, reflux, or ulcers; a good "settling" food after a stomach upset. Super-gentle fiber.
- ❧ Magnesium: works with essential fatty acids, calcium, and the B-complex group to support the nervous system and maintain healthy cell production.
- ❧ Vitamin C, folic acid, vitamin B6, pectin, potassium.

Blackberries

- ❧ Calcium and magnesium; blackberries are especially rich in these, so are good food for the bones.
- ❧ Vitamin C: a cup provides half the recommended daily intake.

Black Currants

- ❧ Antioxidants and B-group vitamins, essential to eye health.
- ❧ Fiber.
- ❧ Vitamin C: a half cup provides more than 100 percent of the daily recommendation for vitamin C.
- ❧ Flavonoids (often found in the same foods that contain vitamin C).

Blueberries

- ❧ Antioxidants and B-group vitamins.
- ❧ Vitamin C.

BERRIES, which have more antioxidants than any other fruits, protect against heart disease, cancer, Alzheimer's, and insomnia, and they reduce inflammation, an underlying factor in age-related diseases. Blueberries help prevent short-term memory loss and lower the risk for breast, oral, and colon cancers in women. Blueberries and cranberries combat urinary tract infections. Tart cherries contain melatonin, which helps you sleep. Go for the whole fruit, not the juice. Add fresh berries to non-fat yogurt. Make a smoothie or toss strawberries or blueberries into a salad. Try to eat a cup of berries every day.

Cantaloupe and Other Melons

- A rich source of carotenoids, which are excellent antioxidants (particularly cantaloupes).
- Flavonoids.

Carambolas (Star Fruit)

- Great eaten straight, like apples, or sliced into fruit salads, blended into fresh fruit juices, or used as a garnish for salads.
- Top-rated for vitamin C.

Cherries

- Beta-carotene: vital for bones and teeth.
- Vitamin C.

Figs

- A "super-food." Delicious in fruit salads. Sweet-tasting dried figs are great alternative to candy. Wonderful chopped into breakfast cereals or eaten as a snack with nuts, seeds, other dried fruit.
- Calcium: good for the bones.
- Fiber: packed with dietary fiber.
- Magnesium.

Grapefruit

- ᷾ Citrus fruits are a rich source of vitamin C and potassium. Pink and red grapefruit varieties are high in beta-carotene.
- ᷾ Flavonoids. Often found in foods that contain vitamin C, flavonoids strengthen capillaries and reduce the risk of bleeding and bruising. Best source: the pith and the zest.

Grapes

- ᷾ Good source of antioxidants, particularly resveratrol, which scientists believe has anti-cancer and cholesterol-lowering properties.

Kiwi Fruit

- ᷾ Very fine source of vitamin C—weight for weight, more than twice that of oranges. One kiwi provides more than 100 percent of the daily recommendation for vitamin C.
- ᷾ Calcium and magnesium: good for the bones.
- ᷾ Fiber.
- ᷾ Small amounts of iron and B vitamins.

ORANGES are the number-one source of vitamin C, the most important water-soluble antioxidant. Besides providing both soluble and insoluble fiber and 170 phytochemicals known to lower the risk for breast cancer, heart disease, and inflammatory conditions in women, they lower the risk of cataracts and premature skin aging. The folate and potassium in citrus are important for women battling high blood pressure whose diuretic medications can cause potassium depletion. Add orange sections to a green salad, perhaps with sliced almonds. They taste great with sweet potatoes. For a healthy dessert, dunk orange sections in melted dark chocolate.

Vegetables

Artichokes

- Natural diuretic and good for the digestion. Contains cyanarin, believed to protect the liver.
- Beta-carotene, folic acid, and most minerals.

Asparagus

- Chock-full of antioxidants, vitamin C, carotene, and folic acid; excellent diuretic that helps rid the body of salt and excess water.
- Chromium: an important factor in balancing blood glucose and blood fats and in protecting the nervous system.
- Beta-carotene: good for the eyes and immune function.
- Vitamin E: prolongs cell life, hastens wound healing, helps reduce scarring.

Avocado

- An excellent skin food. Sadly avoided by many people because they are seen as high in calories and food; avocados should be classified with the "healthy fats" and included more often in the diet.
- Monounsaturates (as in olive oil) and vitamin E.

Bamboo Shoots

- Contain trace elements of vitamin C, calcium, and iron.
- Potassium.

Beans, Green

- Fiber and vitamin C.

Beets

- Fabulous for folate, vitamin C, carotenoids, and potassium.
- Chromium; an important factor in balancing blood glucose and blood fats, and in protecting the nervous system.

GREEN TEA lowers the risk for heart disease, stroke, and breast, colon, and brain cancers. The phytochemicals and possibly the caffeine in green tea also help with weight management. Avoid bottled teas since most health compounds are lost in commercial processing. Brew a pot at home, and aim to drink four cups daily.

Bell Peppers

- Rich in vitamin C, used in the manufacture of collagen, the "glue" that gives skin its elasticity and support; vital for wound healing and protecting against infection.

Brassicas

- An important immune-boosting group that includes Brussels sprouts, all cabbages (including bok choy and red cabbage), Chinese broccoli, green and purple broccoli, calabrese, cauliflower, and kale. Good bone-boosting foods. The stalks, unless too tough, should be sliced up and included in cooking; they are a rich source of minerals. Kale and Chinese broccoli are especially high in calcium.
- Vitamin C: good for the immune system. Some vitamin E, a few B vitamins, folic acid.
- Calcium, magnesium, silica, iron.
- Sulforaphane: an important anti-cancer chemical.
- Plenty of dietary fiber.

Broccoli

- Broccoli stalks are particularly rich in calcium.
- Tiny raw florets used in salads will raise a meal's vitamin C content.
- High scores for sulforaphane, beta-carotene, folate, potassium, magnesium, calcium.

Carrots

- ☞ Contain varying amounts of dietary fiber, beta-carotene, and phenols (sometimes listed as polyphenols)—powerful antioxidant substances that scientists believe may also have immune-boosting properties.
- ☞ Abundant in carotenoids, which include beta-carotene, vital for bones, teeth, eyes, and immune function. Juicing increases the bioavailability of the carotene. Helps support the eyes and boosts the immune system.
- ☞ Small amounts of calcium.

TURMERIC, a main ingredient in curry powder, contains polyphenols, which fight inflammation. A recent study suggested turmeric may have anti-plaque effects that could slow, stop, and perhaps reverse Alzheimer's. It is also linked to improvements in inflammatory bowel disease, ulcerative colitis, colon cancer, pancreatic cancer, breast cancer, psoriasis, and arthritis. Add turmeric to stews and casseroles, or sprinkle it on steamed brown rice, cauliflower, or cabbage.

Celery

- ☞ Vitamin C: a cup of chopped celery provides 10 percent of the daily recommendation.

Dandelion Leaves

- ☞ Natural diuretic.

Garlic

- ☞ Eaten regularly, reduces cholesterol levels and blood viscosity and boosts immunity. Combats infection; has antibacterial properties.
- ☞ Alliums (garlic, onions, leeks, chives) may also block the formation of carcinogenic compounds.
- ☞ Garlic and onions may reduce the risk of thrombosis and hypertension.
- ☞ Raw garlic is more effective than cooked; odor is less strong if used regularly.

- Contains selenium, a trace element now recognized as a vital antioxidant, important not only for a strong immune system, but also for a healthy heart and circulation, and the joints.
- *Tip:* Let garlic sit for 10–15 minutes after chopping and before cooking to allow the active form of phytochemicals (non-nutritive plant chemicals that contain protective, disease-preventing compounds) to develop.

GINGER is as effective as some medications in relieving nausea during pregnancy and after surgery and chemotherapy. It also helps with motion sickness and relieves arthritis. Blend carrots, apples, and a hefty piece of ginger for a spunky juice. Ginger is great when added to a glaze or sauce for salmon, and candied ginger is a delicious addition to a muffin recipe.

Ginger, Fresh Root

- When used as a seasoning, contributes trace amounts of minerals.

Green Vegetables, Leafy

- Because of their antioxidant capabilities, leafy green vegetables are important foods for eye protection, including reducing risk of cataracts and macular degeneration.
- Contains boron, a little-known trace element needed in small amounts but essential for healthy bones and teeth. May be of particular importance in the prevention of osteoporosis and arthritis. Good for the joints.
- Calcium: for healthy blood, blood vessels, skin, bones, and muscle tissue. Calcium works with vitamin C in collagen production. All-important essential fatty acids aren't properly utilized without calcium.
- Magnesium: works with essential fatty acids, calcium, and the B-complex group to support the nervous system and maintain healthy cell production.
- Selenium: antioxidant and anti-inflammatory; supports immune function and improves resistance to infection. Essential for healthy skin, nails, and hair.

- B-complex group of vitamins, for the repair and regeneration of skin tissue, to support the nervous system, and for deriving energy from food—thiamin (B1), riboflavin (B2), niacin (B3), pantothenic acid (B5), pyridoxine (B6), cyanocobalamin (B12), folic acid, and biotin.
- Vitamin C: used in the manufacture of collagen, the "glue" that gives skin its elasticity and support. Vital for wound healing and protecting against infection.
- Vitamin E: prolongs cell life, hastens wound healing, and helps reduce scarring. A vital antioxidant.

Onions

- Contains selenium, a trace element recognized as a vital antioxidant, essential for healthy skin, hair, nails, and hair.

Parsley

- Natural diuretic and digestive aid. All culinary herbs are rich in nutrients.
- Provides an abundance of potassium, folic acid, and carotene.
- Iron: essential for healthy blood.
- Beta-carotene: good for the eyes and immune function.
- Vitamin C.

Potatoes

- Vitamins C, B3, and B6.

Pumpkin

- Beta-carotene: good for the eyes and immune function.

Root vegetables

- Fiber, folic acid, and vitamin C.
- Selenium: antioxidant; anti-inflammatory; supports immune function and improves resistance to infection; essential for healthy skin, hair, and nails.

Spinach

- Because of its antioxidant capabilities, important for eye protection, including reducing risk of cataracts and macular degeneration.
- Magnesium and folic acid. Magnesium is an essential heart nutrient as well as being good for the teeth and bones.
- Beta-carotene: good for the eyes and immune function.

SPINACH prevents birth defects, heart disease, dementia, colon cancer, and vision loss, and protects skin and bones. Full of folate, a B vitamin that prevents birth defects, it also provides lutein, which combats macular degeneration. Spinach helps protect skin from the damaging effects of the sun and helps bones develop. Toss it raw in green salads, or sauté it in olive oil and garlic. Add chopped spinach to your soups, or layer it on crackers or bread with sliced hard-boiled egg and tomato.

Squash, Winter

- ❧ Excellent source of carotenoids.

Sweet Potatoes

- ❧ Loaded with potassium.
- ❧ Beta-carotene: good for the eyes and immune function.

SWEET POTATOES are great for healthy skin. They supply five times the recommended daily value of beta-carotene, which might lower cancer risk, boost defenses against colds and infections, and protect the skin from sun damage. A serving provides more fiber than a slice of whole-wheat bread. Bright orange veggies supply hefty amounts of vitamin C, potassium, and iron. To make fries, slice sweet potatoes into wedges, drizzle with olive oil and salt, and bake at 425 degrees for 15 minutes. Or peel three sweet potatoes, dice and boil until tender, add orange juice concentrate and fresh basil, then drain and food-process until smooth. Or just bake and enjoy.

Tomatoes

- ❧ Particularly rich in vitamin C and lycopene; also some dietary fiber. Recently hailed as an anti-cancer food. Worth eating several times a week.
- ❧ Lycopene (a carotene) is released when tomatoes are cooked and is better absorbed when a little oil is used.
- ❧ Selenium.

TOMATOES are an excellent source of lycopene, an antioxidant that might be a heart saver. According to one study, high blood levels of lycopene could lower heart disease in women by up to 50 percent. Another study suggests it might reduce the risk of fibroid tumors. Since cooked tomatoes contain more lycopene than fresh, choose paste, juice, and sauce. Try to eat seven servings of 1 1/2 tablespoons of tomato paste each week. Add tomato sauce to soups and sauces. To make a mini-pizza, spread tomato sauce on a pita with low-fat cheese and broil.

Watercress

- ❧ Beta-carotene.
- ❧ Vitamin C.

Herbs and Spices

What They Deliver

- ❧ More antioxidants than most fruits and vegetables. Of the fifty foods measured highest in antioxidants, thirteen were herbs and spices. Antioxidants—including beta-carotene, lutein, lycopene, selenium, and vitamins A, C, and E—can protect against heart disease, cancer, and other diseases. Antioxidants are lost when herbs are processed and dried; if you can't grow your own, buy them fresh.

~ Possible role in reducing inflammation, a precursor to such chronic diseases as heart disease, allergies, and Alzheimer's. Not only add flavor but also help heal the body.

Basil

~ Contains ursolic acid, which blocks inflammation, and rosmarinic acid, a powerful antioxidant with therapeutic potential in the treatment or prevention of asthma, ulcers, liver disease, coronary heart disease, cataracts, and cancer.

~ Delicate aroma is produced by essential oils with antibacterial, antifungal, and antioxidant effects.

Cayenne

~ Used in pharmaceuticals to make aspirin.

~ Thought to reduce pain and speed the metabolism.

THE POWER OF SPICES. Researchers are exploring the potential of spices to boost metabolism, promote satiety, aid weight management, and enhance the overall quality of a diet. For example, the capsaicin in peppers is believed to have metabolic-boosting properties. And if the food you eat is flavorful and satisfying, there is a good chance you will eat less and consume fewer calories.

Celery Seed

~ Lowers high blood pressure, heart disease, and cholesterol.

Chamomile

~ Acts as a sedative.

~ Reduces fever.

~ Relieves digestive ailments.

Cilantro

- Also known as Asian parsley or coriander.
- Can reduce high blood sugar and lower levels of cholesterol.
- Can kill dangerous bacteria and help rid the body of toxic metals.

Cinnamon

- Helps control blood sugar levels.
- Combats urinary tract and yeast infections.

Cloves

- Natural anesthetic and antiseptic (due to its eugenol oil); alleviates discomfort and aids in wound healing.
- Combats indigestion and diarrhea.
- Contains antioxidants, which lessen the damage from free radicals, unstable organic molecules that bond with other molecules and are responsible for aging, tissue damage, and possibly some diseases.

Fennel

- Combats colic and gas.
- Diuretic.

Fenugreek

- Eases the symptoms of menopause.
- Relieves constipation.
- Binds with cholesterol in the intestine and encourages the excretion of cholesterol.

Licorice Root

- Relieves symptoms of menopause; in some cases has been shown to be as effective as hormone replacement therapy.

Nutmeg

- Stimulates the cardiovascular system.
- Relieves joint inflammation caused by gout.
- Toxic in large doses. Do not use if pregnant.

Oregano

- ◆ Among the highest in antioxidants of the dried herbs; one study found oregano had 42 times more antioxidants than apples.
- ◆ Relieves respiratory and digestive problems; combats yeast infections.

Parsley

- ◆ Raises the levels of antioxidant enzymes in the blood.
- ◆ Contains high levels of carotenoids; has almost twice the carotenoid content of carrots (the vegetable for which carotenoids were named); matched only by red peppers and kale.

PRACTICING YOUR FRENCH IN THE GARDEN

Plant an outdoor or indoor herb garden. Three savory herbs—basil, parsley, and cilantro—grow equally well in the ground and in pots. All three are rich in disease-fighting, anti-inflammatory phytonutrients (nutrients derived from plant material) and full of antioxidants that build your body's defenses against viruses and disease.

Rosemary

- ◆ Calms the digestive system.
- ◆ Compounds in rosemary appear to help reduce inflammation, a trigger and indirect risk factor for many chronic diseases.
- ◆ Studies are examining its role in heart health.

Saffron

- ◆ Effective in destroying cancer cells found in leukemia.

Sage

- ◆ Combats colds and urinary tract problems.
- ◆ Can be used to treat diabetes.

Thyme

- ❧ Can be crushed and applied to cuts and abrasions as an antiseptic.
- ❧ In tea form, used for colds, menstrual cramps, and to calm the stomach.

Turmeric

- ❧ Combats arthritis and heart disease.
- ❧ Thought to prevent cancer.
- ❧ Researchers are looking into its role in brain health; may protect against cognitive decline associated with aging.

Fish

Fresh Fish

- ❧ Magnesium: magnesium-rich foods are just as important for maintaining healthy muscles, bones, and teeth as calcium; an absolutely essential heart nutrient.
- ❧ Selenium: a vital antioxidant, important not only for a strong immune system, but also for a healthy heart and circulation and joints. Anti-inflammatory; improves resistance to infection; essential for healthy skin, nails, and hair.

Oily Fish

- ❧ Oily fish—especially mackerel, tuna, salmon, and trout—are rich in omega-3 essential fatty acids; EFAs are vital for every cell in the body to function properly, but especially for healthy heart function and circulation; they reduce the stickiness of the blood and help improve the ratio of good cholesterol (high-density lipoproteins, or HDLs).

Salmon

- ❧ Vitamins A and D.
- ❧ Vitamins B1, B2, B3, B5, B6, B12, and biotin.
- ❧ Calcium (canned salmon only) and magnesium: essential heart nutrients as well as being good for the teeth and bones. For healthy blood, blood vessels, skin, bones, and muscle tissue. Calcium works with vitamin C in collagen production. The all-important fatty acids aren't properly utilized without calcium.

- ❧ Omega-3 group of essential fatty acids. Essential fatty acids are important for healthy vision.

SALMON prevents heart disease, depression, and memory loss. It contains omega-3 fats, which reduce the risk for blood clots, boost levels of serotonin, and may lower blood cholesterol. Before cooking, season salmon with salt and pepper, lemon juice, and a drizzle of olive oil; bake in a 350-degree oven for 5 minutes per inch of thickness. Use leftover pieces in a green salad, or spread a cracker with Dijon mustard, leftover salmon, and capers. Aim to eat two 4-oz. servings each week.

Mackerel

- ❧ Calcium (canned mackerel only) and magnesium. Essential heart nutrients as well as good for teeth and bones. For healthy blood, blood vessels, skin, bones, and muscle tissue. Calcium works with vitamin C in collagen production. The all-important fatty acids aren't properly utilized without calcium.
- ❧ Zinc (canned mackerel only): immune-boosting and essential for healthy skin.
- ❧ Omega-3 group of essential fatty acids, important for healthy sight.

Shellfish

- ❧ Chromium: an important factor in balancing blood glucose and blood fats.
- ❧ Selenium.
- ❧ Zinc: for wound healing and healthy growth and repair of cells.

Cereals (Grains)

What They Deliver

- ❧ B-complex group and vitamin E.
- ❧ Chromium, magnesium, and selenium.

Millet

- ⮞ Zinc: for wound healing and healthy growth and repair of cells.

Oats

- ⮞ Good source of soluble fiber, which may help reduce cholesterol.
- ⮞ Vitamin B.
- ⮞ Small amounts of vitamins B2, B3, B6, and folic acid.
- ⮞ Zinc: for wound healing, healthy growth and repair of cells.

Wheat

- ⮞ Good source of soluble fiber, which may help reduce cholesterol.
- ⮞ Contains large quantities of manganese, phosphorus, magnesium, and selenium.
- ⮞ Rich in zinc, copper, iron, and potassium.
- ⮞ Rich in vitamins B1, B2, B3, B5, B6, and B9.
- ⮞ Reduces risk of high blood pressure, diabetes, and high cholesterol.

Corn

- ⮞ Rich in phosphorus, magnesium, manganese, zinc, copper, iron, and selenium.
- ⮞ Vitamins B1, B2, B3, B6, and B9.

OLD-FASHIONED OATMEAL helps maintain a healthy weight. Its combination of fiber and water fills you up on fewer calories and digests slowly. A soluble fiber called glucan, available in oatmeal when it's mixed with liquid, forms as a viscous gel that helps lower risk for diabetes and heart disease. Enjoy in the morning with chopped apples, cinnamon, and nuts, which add staying power (satiation) because of their healthy fats.

Rice (Brown)

- ◦ Essential fatty acids.
- ◦ Magnesium: as important as calcium for maintaining healthy muscles, bones, and teeth.
- ◦ Selenium and zinc.
- ◦ Many times more nourishing than white rice; an excellent source of potassium, vitamin B3, vitamin E, and folic acid.
- ◦ Gentle but effective dietary fiber.

Rye

- ◦ Zinc: for wound healing and healthy growth and repair of cells.

WHEAT GERM is a gold mine of nutrition. A half cup supplies more than half of a woman's daily need for magnesium, which is essential for reducing stress, building bones, and regulating thyroid function— yet three out of four women don't get enough of it. Consuming a magnesium-rich diet cuts the risk of diabetes by 48 percent. Sprinkle it on yogurt or oatmeal, add to it pancake and muffin batter, or blend it with peanut butter.

Beans and Legumes

What They Deliver

- ◦ B-complex group of vitamins: for repair and regeneration of skin tissue, to support the nervous system, and for deriving energy from food—thiamin (B1), riboflavin (B2), niacin (B3), pantothenic acid (B5), pyridoxine (B6), cyanocobalamin (B12), folic acid, and biotin.
- ◦ Iron: essential for healthy blood.
- ◦ Magnesium: magnesium-rich foods such as legumes are as important as calcium for maintaining healthy muscles, bones, and teeth. Works with

essential fatty acids, calcium, and the B-complex group to support the nervous system and maintain healthy cell production.

꙰ Vitamin B2.

꙰ Zinc: immune-boosting and essential for maintaining healthy skin.

BLACK BEANS are a great food if you want to manage your weight, avoid heart disease, and maintain healthy bowels. Cholesterol free and almost fat free, they are rich in fiber and nutrients: A serving supplies more than a half day's requirement of folic acid, plus hefty amounts of calcium, magnesium, iron, and zinc. Use rinsed, canned beans in salads and soups, or warm them, sprinkle with cilantro, and serve over brown rice.

Garbanzo Beans (Chickpeas)

꙰ Zinc: immune-boosting and essential for maintaining healthy skin.

Lentils

꙰ Zinc: immune-boosting and essential for maintaining healthy skin.

Peas

꙰ Vitamin C and folic acid.

꙰ Fiber and small amounts of iron, zinc, and magnesium.

Red Kidney Beans

꙰ Zinc: immune-boosting and essential for maintaining healthy skin.

Soybeans

꙰ Calcium: for healthy blood, blood vessels, skin, bones, and muscle tissue. The all-important fatty acids aren't properly utilized without calcium.

꙰ Thought by some to help balance the hormones.

꙰ Good source of phytoestrogens, which may help reduce the risk of breast and prostate cancer.

> ❧ Tofu (bean curd) is an excellent protein source for vegetarians—rich in calcium, magnesium, iron, and some vitamin E.

Dairy Products

> ❧ Use in moderation and choose organic products when possible.

Butter

> ❧ Vitamin A: good for the eyes.

Buttermilk

> ❧ Calcium.

Cheese

> ❧ Calcium and vitamin B2.
> ❧ Vitamin A: good for the eyes.
> ❧ Zinc: for wound healing and healthy growth and repair of cells.

Eggs

> ❧ Protein.
> ❧ Chromium: an important factor in balancing blood glucose and blood fats and protecting the nervous system.
> ❧ Selenium and small amounts of iron and zinc.
> ❧ Vitamin A: good for the eyes.
> ❧ Vitamin B2.
> ❧ Some vitamin B3, B12, D, E, and folic acid.
> ❧ Choose organic, vegetarian-fed, omega-3 eggs.

Yogurt

> ❧ Calcium.
> ❧ Yogurt with live and active cultures is beneficial not only to the digestion but also to the gut generally, as a valuable source of friendly bacteria.
> ❧ Provides easily digestible protein, magnesium, potassium, zinc, vitamins B1, and B2, and vitamin A.

YOGURT provides calcium, which protects against osteoporosis. It encourages the growth of healthy bacteria in the digestive tract and so lowers the risk of disorders ranging from diarrhea to certain allergies; it eases the symptoms of lactose intolerance and irritable bowel syndrome, and may help prevent colorectal cancer. The best source for high levels of bacteria is plain yogurt. Sweeten it with fresh fruit, and use it in smoothies and as a fruit topping.

Nuts

What They Deliver

- All contain potassium, magnesium, selenium, iron, and zinc. Valuable also for their dietary fiber and monounsaturated and polyunsaturated fatty-acid content. For best nourishment value, purchase them fresh and unbroken, not salted, crushed, or roasted.
- B-complex group. For the repair and regeneration of skin tissue, to support the nervous system, and for the release of energy from food.
- Calcium: for healthy blood, blood vessels, skin, bones, and muscle tissue; calcium works with vitamin C in collagen production.
- Iron: essential for healthy blood.
- Zinc: for wound healing and healthy growth and repair of cells.

Almonds

- Calcium and magnesium.
- Omega-6 essential fatty acids.
- Potassium, selenium, iron, and zinc.

Brazil Nuts

- Calcium and magnesium.
- Omega-6 essential fatty acids.
- Potassium, selenium, iron, and zinc.

    ❧ Valuable also for their dietary fiber and monounsaturated and polyunsaturated fatty-acid content.

Cashew Nuts

    ❧ Potassium.

Hazelnuts

    ❧ Boron.
    ❧ Potassium, magnesium, iron, and zinc.
    ❧ Valuable also for their dietary fiber and monounsaturated and polyunsaturated fatty acid content.

Macadamia Nuts

    ❧ Potassium and iron.
    ❧ Valuable also for their dietary fiber and monounsaturated and polyunsaturated fatty-acid content.

Walnuts

    ❧ Omega-3 essential fatty acids.

Seeds

What They Deliver

    ❧ Edible seeds include pumpkin, sesame, sunflower, linseeds, flax, chia, poppy, celery, dill, fennel, and fenugreek. Rich in essential fatty acids. Provide zinc, potassium, magnesium, and iron. Sunflower seeds are particularly good for vitamin E. Sesame seeds are high in calcium.
    ❧ The B-complex group of vitamins for the repair and regeneration of skin tissue, to support the nervous system, and for deriving energy from food—thiamin (B1), riboflavin (B2), niacin (B3), pantothenic acid (B5), pyridoxine (B6), cyanocobalamin (B12), folic acid, biotin.
    ❧ Calcium: for healthy blood, blood vessels, skin, bones, and muscle tissue; works with vitamin C in collagen production.
    ❧ Iron: essential for healthy blood.
    ❧ Vitamin E: prolongs cell life, hastens wound healing, and helps reduce scarring. A vital antioxidant.
    ❧ Zinc: for wound healing, healthy growth, and repair of cells.

CHOCOLATE is derived from the seed of the tropical *Theobroma cacao* tree. A serving of dark chocolate (at least 70 percent cocoa powder) measures 9,000 units on the ORAC (oxygen radical absorption capacity) scale, compared to the average of 2,000 units found in servings of most fruit and vegetables. Dark chocolate is thought to lower heart disease by an estimated 20 percent by reducing total cholesterol, inhibiting blood clots and artery inflammation, and keeping arteries elastic.

Linseeds and Flaxseeds

- Rich in essential fatty acids. Contain zinc, potassium, magnesium, and iron.

Pumpkin Seeds

- Essential fatty acids.
- Potassium, magnesium, and iron.
- Zinc: an immune-building essential.

Sesame Seeds

- For healthy blood, blood vessels, skin, bones, and muscle tissue. The all-important fatty acids aren't properly utilized without calcium.
- Vitamin E: prolongs cell life, hastens wound healing, and helps reduce scarring; a vital antioxidant.
- Rich in essential fatty acids. Contain small amounts of magnesium, phosphorus, and iron.

Sunflower Seeds

- Rich in essential fatty acids. Also high in zinc, potassium, magnesium, vitamins B3 and B6, and folic acid.
- Especially good for vitamin E.

Oils

Almond Oil

- ❧ Omega-6 essential fatty acid.

Cold-pressed Oils

- ❧ Cold-pressed oils are those such as sunflower, sesame, walnut, extra-virgin olive oil, safflower, soybean, coconut, and linseed oil. Most mass-produced cooking oils are processed and refined using heat and solvents. Cold pressing, a more expensive method, retains more of the natural goodness of the oil, in particular the essential fatty acids.
- ❧ Polyunsaturated oils tend to be less stable when heated; use them for salads and light cooking. Extra-virgin olive oil is predominately monounsaturated and more stable at higher temperatures, although frying impairs the flavor. Try to include a tablespoon of cold-pressed unrefined oil to the diet every day. Refrigerate to keep them fresh.
- ❧ Vitamin E: hastens wound healing and helps reduce scarring.

Fish Oils

- ❧ Rich in omega-3 essential fatty acids: vital for good muscle tone, healthy hair, strong nails, hormone production, and healthy skin.
- ❧ Vitamin A–rich fish oils, such as cod liver oil, are excellent for the eyes, help to protect cell membranes, and may reduce the risk of glaucoma.
- ❧ Vitamin D.

Olive Oil (Extra Virgin)

- ❧ Rich in monounsaturates. The best choice of oil for cooking; although frying impairs its flavor. Also makes delicious salad dressings. ❧

Notes

(p. 2)   *. . . 137.6 pounds:* msnbc.msn.com/id/11149568/ns/health-fitness/t/ french-are-getting-taller-fatter/ (accessed Oct. 15, 2011).

(p. 2)   *. . . 164.7 pounds:* Margaret A. McDowell et al., "Anthropometric Reference Data for Children and Adults: United States, 2003–2006," *National Health Statistics Reports*, no. 10 (Oct. 22, 2008); www.cdc.gov/nchs/fastats/bodymeas.htm (accessed Oct. 15, 2011).

(p. 3)   *Did someone say croissant?:* infoplease.com/world/statistics/life-expectancy-country-2009.html (accessed Oct. 15, 2011).

(p. 4)   *. . . 10.5 percent of the French population is obese:* www.oecd.org/dataoecd/55/2/44117530.pdf (accessed Oct. 17, 2011), p. 57. Cited in David R. Bassett Jr., "Pedometer-Measured Physical Activity and Health Behaviors in U.S. Adults," *Medicine & Science in Sports & Exercise*, vol. 42, no. 10 (Oct. 2010), pp. 1819–25.

(p. 11)   *. . . level of satisfaction with their bodies:* Emily A. Hamilton et al., "Predictors of Media Effects on Body Dissatisfaction in European American Women," *Sex Roles*, vol. 56, nos. 5–6 (2007), pp. 397–402. Reported in: www.sciencedaily.com/releases/2007/03/070326152704. htm (accessed Oct. 15, 2011).

(p. 13)   . . . *exercise-induced weight loss:* L. P. Svetkey et al., "Comparison of Strategies for Sustaining Weight Loss: The Weight Loss Maintenance Randomized Controlled Trial," *Journal of the American Medical Association*, vol. 299, no. 10 (2008), pp. 1139–48; W. Yang et al., "Genetic Epidemiology of Obesity," *Epidemiological Reviews*, vol. 29, no. 1 (2007), pp. 49–61; T. Rankinen et al., "The Human Obesity Gene Map: The 2005 Update," *Obesity*, vol. 14, no. 4 (2006), pp. 529–644; www.iotf.org/aboutobesity.asp.

(p. 13)   . . . *periods of over-eating, or bingeing:* E. Saltzman and S. B. Roberts, "The Role of Energy Expenditure in Energy Regulation: Findings from a Decade of Research," *Nutrition Reviews*, vol. 53, no. 8 (1995), pp. 209–220; N. S. Burgess, "Effect of a Very-Low Calorie Diet on Body Composition and Resting Metabolic Rate in Obese Men and Women," *Journal of the American Dietetic Association*, vol. 91, no. 4 (1991), pp. 430–34; P. J. Rogers, "Eating Habits and Appetite Control: A Psychobiological Perspective," *Proceedings of the Nutrition Society*, vol. 58, no. 1 (1999), pp. 59–67.

(p. 13)   *One study . . . :* C. K. Martin et al., "Effect of Calorie Restriction on Resting Metabolic Rate and Spontaneous Physical Activity," *Obesity*, vol. 15, no. 12 (Dec. 2007), pp. 2964–73.

(p. 13)   . . . *and another . . . :* L. M. Redman et al. "Metabolic and Behavioral Compensations in Response to Caloric Restriction: Implications for the Maintenance of Weight Loss." *PLoS ONE*, vol. 4, no. 2 (Feb. 9, 2009).

(p. 16)   . . . *when to stop eating:* Cornell Food & Brand Lab (2008, Feb. 18), "Why Don't the French Get as Fat as Americans? Americans Eat Until the TV Show Is Over," *Science Daily*, www.sciencedaily.com/releases/2008/02/080215103153.htm; Brian Wansink et al., "Internal and External Cues of Meal Cessation: The French Paradox Redux?" *Obesity*, vol. 15, no. 12 (2007), pp. 2920–24.

(p. 17)   . . . *a variety of harmful conditions:* Meghan A.T.B. Reese, "Underweight: A Heavy Concern," *Today's Dietitian*, vol. 10, no. 1 (Jan. 2008), p. 56, www.todaysdietitian.com/newarchives/tdjan2008pg56.shtml (accessed Oct. 15, 2011).

(p. 32)   . . . *is very similar:* V. Hainer et al., "A Twin Study of Weight Loss and Metabolic Efficiency," *International Journal of Obesity*, vol. 25, no. 4 (2001), pp. 533–37.

(p. 42)   . . . *all the benefits it's capable of:* J. C. Rickman et al., "Nutritional Comparison of Fresh, Frozen and Canned Fruits and Vegetables. Part I. Vitamins C and B and Phenolic Compounds," *Journal of the Science of Food and Agriculture,* 87 (2007), pp. 930–44; J. C. Rickman et al., "Nutritional Comparison of Fresh, Frozen and Canned Fruits and Vegetables. Part II. Vitamin A and Carotenoids, Vitamin E, Minerals and Fiber," *Journal of the Science of Food and Agriculture,* 87 (2007), pp. 1185–96. Both reported in: www.acefitness.org/blog/859/?DCMP=RSSask-the-expert (accessed Oct. 15, 2011).

(p. 46)   ". . . *It's sad":* Elaine Sciolino, "Sans Makeup, S'il Vous Plaît," *New York Times,* May 25, 2006, www.nytimes.com/2006/05/25/fashion/thursdaystyles/25skin.html?ei=5087&en=c77268d31d7f6f34&ex=1148788800&pagewanted=all

(p. 47)   . . . *three times per day:* W. J. Cunliffe et al., "A Double-blind Trial of a Zinc Sulphate/Citrate Complex and Tetracycline in the Treatment of Acne Vulgaris," *British Journal of Dermatology,* vol. 101, no. 3 (Sept. 1979), pp. 321–25.

(p. 57)   *In an international study . . . :* P. Rozin et al., "Attitudes to Food and the Role of Food in Life in the U.S.A., Japan, Flemish Belgium and France: Possible Implications for the Diet–Health Debate," *Appetite,* vol. 33, no. 2 (Oct. 1999), pp. 163–80.

(p. 58)   . . . *the absorption of iron from a meal:* Christopher K. Rayner and Michael Horowitz, "Food That Tastes Good Is More Nutritious," *Tufts University Health and Nutrition Letter,* vol. 18, no. 8 (Oct. 2000), p. 1.

(p. 70)   . . . *a weight-loss strategy:* "HCG Diet: Look Elsewhere for Weight Loss," www.dietsinreview.com/diet_column/07/hcg-diet-look-elsewhere-for-weight-loss/#ixzz0t0uDA5VV (accessed Oct. 15, 20110).

(p. 71)   . . . *greater levels of abdominal fat:* M. Ebrecht et al., "Perceived Stress and Cortisol Levels Predict Speed of Wound Healing in Healthy Male Adults," *Psychoneuroendocrinology,* vol. 29, no. 6 (July 2004), pp. 798–809.

(p. 72)   . . . *like heart attacks and diabetes:* T. Chandola et al., "Chronic Stress at Work and the Metabolic Syndrome: Prospective Study," *British Medical Journal,* vol. 332 (2006).

(p. 72)   *. . . and exercise physiologist:* S. Reinberg, "Low-Cal Diets May Make You *Gain* Weight," healthfinder.gov, Apr. 8, 2010, news.healingwell.com/index.php?p=news1&id=637842 (accessed Oct. 16, 2011).

(p. 75)   *. . . online magazine* The Morning News: themorningnews.org/archives/personalities/roundtable_the_french_paradox.php (accessed Oct. 16, 2011).

(p. 79)   *. . . 13 percent of the U.S. Gross National Product:* Caroline McColloch, "The Industrialization of Food, *Dayton Nutrition Examiner*, Oct. 23, 2009, examiner.com/nutrition-in-dayton/the-industrialization-of-food (accessed Oct. 16, 2011).

(p. 79)   *. . . entire academic departments:* Department of Health and Human Services, *The Surgeon General's Report on Nutrition and Health*, Washington, D.C. (1988).

(p. 81)   *. . . Rossen reports:* Courtney Drewsen, *Dallas Fitness Examiner*, June 16, 2010, examiner.com/fitness-in-dallas/frozen-meal-labels-are-not-what-they-seem (accessed Oct. 16, 2011).

(p. 81)   *. . . the same goes for the fat content:* "NBC's *Today* Show Utilizes EMSL Analytical's Food Testing Laboratory," WebWire, June 17, 2010, www.webwire.com/ViewPressRel.asp?aId=118739 (accessed Oct. 16, 2011).

(p. 84)   *. . . to damage your health:* D. Mozaffarian et al., "Trans Fatty Acids and Cardiovascular Disease," *New England Journal of Medicine*, vol. 354, no. 15 (Apr. 13, 2006), pp. 1601–13.

(p. 86)   *. . . cannot tolerate aspartame:* R. Blaylock, *Excitotoxins: The Taste That Kills.* Santa Fe, NM: Health Press, 1996.

(p. 87)   *. . . the study, published in* Behavioral Neuroscience, *noted:* Susan E. Swithers and Terry L. Davidson, "A Role for Sweet Taste: Calorie Predictive Relations in Energy Regulation by Rats," *Behavioral Neuroscience,* vol. 122, no. 1 (2008), pp. 161–73.

(p. 87)   *. . . by overdoing it:* W. Pierce et al. "Overeating by Young Obesity-Prone and Lean Rats Caused by Tastes Associated with Low-Energy Foods," *Obesity,* vol. 15, no. 8 (Aug. 2007).

(p. 88)   *. . . hyperactivity levels rose dramatically:* D. McCann et al., "Food Additives and Hyperactive Behavior in 3-Year-Old and 8/9-Year-Old Children in the Community: A Randomized, Double-Blinded, Placebo-

Controlled Trial," *The Lancet*, vol. 370, no. 9598 (Nov. 3, 2007), pp. 1560–67.

(p. 93)   . . . *like a good chardonnay:* Judith Weintraub, "The Fall and Rise of French Bread," *Washington Post*, Aug. 24, 2005. www.washingtonpost. com/wp-dyn/content/article/2005/08/23/AR2005082300291.html (accessed Oct. 16, 2011).

(p. 99)   . . . *University of California, San Diego:* Alain Sailhac et al., *The French Culinary Institute's Salute to Healthy Cooking*, New York: St. Martin's/ Rodale, 1998, p. 2.

(p. 99)   ". . . *Americans eat just three":* Ibid., pp. 3, 4.

(p. 100)   ". . . *conferring this benefit":* Ibid., p. 7.

(p. 100)   . . . *because it contains flavonoids:* Janet Raloff, "Grape Juice: Better Than Aspirin"? *Science News Online*, Mar. 22, 1997, www.sciencenews.org/ sn_arc97/3_22_97/food.htm (accessed Oct. 16, 2011).

(p. 100)   ". . . *are powerful antioxidants":* Sailhac et al., *The French Culinary Institute's Salute to Healthy Cooking*, pp. 9–10.

(p. 107)   . . . *more lean muscle mass:* R. Ferraro et al., "Lower Sedentary Metabolic Rate in Women Compared with Men," *Journal of Clinical Investigation*, vol. 90, no. 3 (Sept. 1992), pp. 780–84.

(p. 116)   . . . *in the* Annals of Internal Medicine: Arlet V. Nedeltcheva et al., "Insufficient Sleep Undermines Dietary Efforts to Reduce Adiposity," *Annals of Internal Medicine*, vol. 153, no. 7 (Oct. 5, 2010), pp. 435–41.

(p. 119)   ". . . *obesity rates above 25 percent":* F as in Fat: How Obesity Threatens America's Future 2010, Trust for America's Health, Robert Wood Johnson Foundation, 2010. Reported in: businessweek.com/lifestyle/ content/healthday/640650.html (accessed Oct. 16, 2011).

(p. 121)   . . . *a new chemotherapy treatment:* Brenda O'Regan and Thomas Hurley, "Placebo: The Hidden Asset in Healing," *Investigations: The Institute of Noetic Sciences Research Bulletin*, vol. 2, no. 14 (1985).

(p. 124)   . . . *even a punishment:* "Mental Health Benefits of Exercise," FindCounseling.com, www.findcounseling.com/journal/health-fitness/ (accessed Oct. 16, 2011).

(p. 127)   ". . . *both physical and mental health":* American Psychological Association, "Excessive Exercise Can Be Addicting, New Study

Says," *ScienceDaily* (Aug. 18, 2009), www.sciencedaily.com/releases/2009/08/090817143600.htm (accessed Oct. 16, 2011).

(p. 132) *... and Japan (7,168)*: David R. Bassett Jr., "Pedometer-Measured Physical Activity and Health Behaviors in U.S. Adults," *Medicine & Science in Sports & Exercise*, vol. 42, no. 10 (Oct. 2010), pp. 1819–25. Reported in: www.post-gazette.com/pg/10298/1097522-114.stm (accessed Oct. 16, 2011).

(p. 133) *... less likely to develop it:* Susan B. Sisson et al., "Accelerometer-Determined Steps/Day and Metabolic Syndrome," *American Journal of Preventive Medicine,* vol. 38, no. 6 (June 2010), pp. 575–82.

(p. 133) *... intrigued me:* K. I. Erickson et al., "Physical Activity Predicts Gray Matter Volume in Late Adulthood: The Cardiovascular Health Study," *Neurology*, vol. 75 (Oct. 19, 2010), pp. 1415–22. Reported in: news.discovery.com/human/take-a-walk-to-protect-your-memory.html (accessed Oct. 16, 2011).

(p. 162) *... the Loire Valley of France:* "French Paradox in the School Cafeteria"? Healthy Schools Campaign, May 14, 1997, healthyschoolscampaign.typepad.com/healthy_schools_campaign/international_forum/ (accessed Oct. 16, 2011).

(p. 163) *... comfortably positioned at the table:* Deborah Madison, "School Lunch Abroad: Another Way to Eat," *Culinate*, Sept. 6, 2007, www.culinate.com/search/q,vt=top,q=school+lunch+abroad/32924 (accessed Oct. 16, 2001).

(p. 166) *"... a spark plug":* "Progress Report on "Let's Move!'," NACS Online, http://www.nacsonline.com/NACS/News/Daily/Pages/ND0209112.aspx (accessed Nov. 1, 2011).

(p. 174) *... criteria for bulimia nervosa:* David S. Rosen, "Identification and Management of Eating Disorders in Children and Adolescents," *Pediatrics,* vol. 126, no. 6 (Dec. 2010), pp. 1240–53.

(p. 175) *... an increase of 118 percent:* Evelyn Attia and B. Timothy Walsh, "Behavioral Management for Anorexia Nervosa," *New England Journal of Medicine,* vol. 360, no. 5 (2009) pp. 500–506.

Mini-Index

About the Author

Carol Cottrill, CNC, worked in the film business for nearly twenty years, first as a principal actor in television commercials, then as an agent for film directors. In the late 1990s, at the pinnacle of her career—while attending the Cannes Film Festival, no less—she decided to switch fields entirely. She set out in pursuit of a degree in nutrition.

Carol's desire to learn more about food and its role in a healthy lifestyle was sparked by a two-year stint with an overzealous fitness trainer who talked her into a low-carb regimen. What began as an innocent attempt to improve her diet and fitness level ended in unwarranted restrictive eating and extreme exercise.

Through her studies in holistic nutrition, Carol began to unravel America's unhealthy preoccupation with food and exercise. In 2001 she earned a Bachelor of Science degree in holistic nutrition from Clayton College of Natural Health, where she graduated with highest honors. That same year, she opened a private nutritional practice in Atlanta. It has since become Carol's mission to expose the futility of serial dieting and the damage and distress it causes for millions of women.

Born in Pittsburgh, Carol has lived on both coasts, and she recently settled in New York City with her husband, John, and their two dogs. She is a seasoned overseas traveler; her visits to Europe have opened her eyes to the way other cultures eat—routinely enjoying the best foods, even those considered "decadent," while staying healthy and controlling weight.

Carol divides her time between her Manhattan and central Florida offices, counseling clients who include celebrities from the worlds of fashion, music, medicine, and business. A regular speaker on subjects ranging from the dangers of fad dieting to osteoporosis, she enjoys expressing her views in articles for magazines and newspapers, including the *San Francisco Chronicle* and the *New York Post*. She is an expert for Dr. Mehmet Oz's interactive social Q&A platform, Sharecare.com. Carol also contributes to a variety of popular websites and blogs and regularly posts to several social networks.

In pursuing her specialty, weight management, Carol targets the disordered eating that results from the American obsession with being thin. With wit and wisdom, she engages us in a new conversation about the importance of eating authentic, high-quality food, and the roles that pleasure and balance play in proper nutrition and maintaining a healthy weight.

BUY A SHARE OF THE FUTURE IN YOUR COMMUNITY

These certificates make great holiday, graduation and birthday gifts that can be personalized with the recipient's name. The cost of one S.H.A.R.E. or one square foot is $54.17. The personalized certificate is suitable for framing and will state the number of shares purchased and the amount of each share, as well as the recipient's name. The home that you participate in "building" will last for many years and will continue to grow in value.

Here is a sample SHARE certificate:

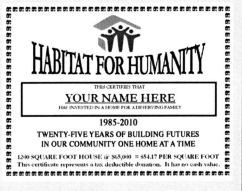

THIS CERTIFIES THAT

YOUR NAME HERE

HAS INVESTED IN A HOME FOR A DESERVING FAMILY

1985-2010

TWENTY-FIVE YEARS OF BUILDING FUTURES
IN OUR COMMUNITY ONE HOME AT A TIME

1200 SQUARE FOOT HOUSE @ $65,000 = $54.17 PER SQUARE FOOT
This certificate represents a tax deductible donation. It has no cash value.

YES, I WOULD LIKE TO HELP!

I support the work that Habitat for Humanity does and I want to be part of the excitement! As a donor, I will receive periodic updates on your construction activities but, more importantly, I know my gift will help a family in our community realize the dream of homeownership. **I would like to SHARE in your efforts against substandard housing in my community!** *(Please print below)*

PLEASE SEND ME _____ SHARES at $54.17 EACH = $ $_____

In Honor Of: _____

Occasion: (Circle One)   HOLIDAY   BIRTHDAY   ANNIVERSARY

      OTHER: _____

Address of Recipient: _____

Gift From: _____ *Donor Address:* _____

Donor Email: _____

I AM ENCLOSING A CHECK FOR $ $_____ PAYABLE TO HABITAT FOR HUMANITY <u>OR</u> PLEASE CHARGE MY VISA OR MASTERCARD *(CIRCLE ONE)*

Card Number _____ Expiration Date: _____

Name as it appears on Credit Card _____ Charge Amount $ _____

Signature _____

Billing Address _____

Telephone # Day _____ Eve _____

PLEASE NOTE: Your contribution is tax-deductible to the fullest extent allowed by law.
Habitat for Humanity • P.O. Box 1443 • Newport News, VA 23601 • 757-596-5553
www.HelpHabitatforHumanity.org

CPSIA information can be obtained at www.ICGtesting.com
Printed in the USA
BVOW02s1158051113

335502BV00007B/169/P